Contents

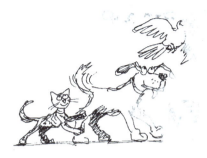

Perfect your portfolio

Lorraine Allan and Margaret Blezard

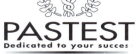

PASTEST
Dedicated to your success

© 2004 PasTest
Egerton Court
Parkgate Estate
Knutsford
Cheshire
WA16 8DX

Telephone: 01565 752000

Published 2004

ISBN: 1 904627 28 5

A catalogue record for this book is available from the British Library.

The information contained within this book was obtained by the authors from reliable sources. However, while every effort has been made to ensure its accuracy, no responsibility for loss, damage or injury occasioned to any person acting or refraining from action as a result of information contained herein can be accepted by the publishers or authors.

PasTest Revision Books and Intensive Courses

PasTest has been established in the field of postgraduate medical education since 1972, providing revision books and intensive study courses for doctors preparing for their professional examinations. Books and courses are available for the following specialties:

MRCGP, MRCP Part 1 and 2, MRCPCH Part 1 and 2, MRCPsych, MRCS, MRCOG, DRCOG, DCH, FRCA, PLAB.

For further details contact:

PasTest, Freepost, Knutsford, Cheshire WA16 7BR
Tel: 01565 752000 Fax: 01565 650264
www.pastest.co.uk enquiries@pastest.co.uk

Text prepared by Vision Typesetting Ltd, Manchester
Printed and bound in Great Britain by Page Bros (Norwich) Ltd

About the authors

Lorraine Allan BVSc MRCVS PGCE D32/33/34
Qualified from Liverpool University in 1975 and has taught
Veterinary Nursing at Myerscough College for many years.
Currently she is course tutor for both the BSc (Hons) Veterinary
Nursing and BSc(Hons) Clinical Veterinary Nursing courses and
works closely with the Myerscough VNAC team as BSc Internal
Verifier.

Margaret Blezard CertEd. VN D32/33/34/35
Level 2 Course Tutor and Veterinary Nursing Lecturer at
Myerscough College in Preston. She was originally involved with
the inception of the current NVQ scheme firstly as an assessor in
practice, working with the original consultation process and then
as one of the first External Verifiers for the RCVS.

Acknowledgements

Special thanks to Kathy Kissick, the Myerscough Veterinary Nursing and VNAC teams. Not forgetting our many students and their assessors, without whose contributions this book would never have been written.

Also grateful thanks to the RCVS External Verifiers, for their help and advice.

Foreword

To many student veterinary nurses and, indeed, to many VN assessors the word 'portfolio' engenders a mild panic. The level 2 and level 3 portfolios are seen as something to sweat over, swear at and generally have a miserable time with until they are completed. The general view appears to be that they are distinct from the VN course and even detract from the 'real studying'. The reason for that seems to be a lack of understanding of the objectives of the portfolios and a distinct lack of guidance as to their completion.

Perfect your portfolio takes you through levels 2 and 3: from the very first stages of explaining 'NVQ-speak', to final preparations prior to sending them for assessment.

This book not only helps the student to feel more confident about their portfolio; it also explains how completion of the portfolio can be a very good learning tool. Suggestions of suitable cases, how to make the most of appendices, where and when to cross-reference and examples of completed log sheets are set out in plain English in a very easy-to-read style. Handy, practical advice is given throughout, including a useful 'what if' chapter devoted to specific advice for 'portfolio emergencies.'

This book is a 'must have' for any VN student and Assessor.

Julian G Hoad BSc(Hons) BVetMed MRCVS

Introduction

Your portfolio is the perfect way to demonstrate practical veterinary nursing skills and show your huge commitment to NVQ VN training achievement.

This book was written at the instigation of and for the benefit of student veterinary nurses and their assessors. Its aims are to:

* Provide an insight into successful portfolio compilation

* Reduce the workload of both student and assessor

* Answer commonly asked questions regarding the portfolio and assessment process

* Make NVQ terminology understandable.

Quite a task, but here we go!!

The Royal College of Veterinary Surgeons (RCVS) introduced the first training and assessment programme in veterinary nursing, in 1961. Since then radical changes have been implemented in veterinary nursing training. The implementation of a National Vocational Qualification (NVQ) in Veterinary Nursing in January 1999 provided a milestone, with the introduction of a national benchmark to standardise the quality of veterinary nursing care and training.

To achieve the Veterinary Nursing qualification and become a Listed Veterinary Nurse it is necessary to attain the following:

* NVQ Level 2 This includes attaining the Level 2 RCVS external written examinations and successfully completing the Level 2 portfolio.

* NVQ Level 3. This includes attaining the Level 3 RCVS external

written and practical/oral examinations, and successfully
completing the Level 3 portfolio.

* Fulfil RCVS regulatory requirements in terms of work-based
experience.

This book, however, concentrates on helping to fulfil the Levels 2 and
3 portfolio requirements.

We have consulted a large number of students and qualified
veterinary nurses, many of whom are assessors, for their opinions as
to the contents of this book. This is what we have concluded is
necessary to explain how to make portfolio compilation relatively
painless. If it fulfils your needs please inform your friends and
colleagues; if not, then contact us and we will endeavour to
encompass your needs in the next edition.

Essential terminology

We have tried to keep NVQ terminology to a minimum, as we are
aware that this can be a major turn-off for the vast majority of
student veterinary nurses (and assessors), but it is important that
some terms are understood to facilitate completion of the
portfolio. **Remember that at the beginning of your course, when
you had to come to terms with veterinary terminology, it was just
as confusing.**

Assessment – This is the process of collecting evidence and
making judgements as to whether the performance criteria and
scope have been met.

Assessor – Pivotal to the assessment process, the assessor is the
person responsible for ensuring that the correct level of skill,
knowledge and understanding has been achieved. The assessor
must be a listed veterinary nurse or veterinary surgeon who holds
the appropriate Training and Development Lead Body (TDLB)
qualifications D32/33 or the new equivalent A1.

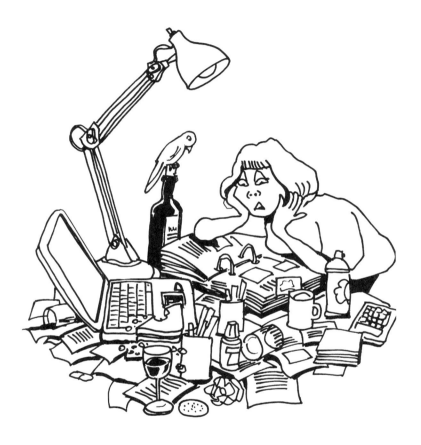

This book will help take the stress out of preparing your portfolio.

Award – A general term for that which is given to an individual in recognition of the attainment of an NVQ qualification.

Awarding Body – A body approved by the Qualifications and Curriculum Authority (QCA) for the purpose of awarding NVQs. In the case of veterinary nursing this is the Royal College of Veterinary Surgeons (RCVS).

Candidate – An individual undertaking an NVQ qualification route – in this instance the student veterinary nurse.

Certificate – A document issued to an individual by an awarding body formally signifying the attainment of an NVQ or a unit of competence.

Competence – The ability to perform to the standards required in employment.

Evidence Gatherer – A person who does not hold an assessor qualification but is suitably qualified and competent to assess performance and provide a witness statement. However, a qualified assessor must verify this.

External Verifier – A person appointed by the awarding body (RCVS), whose responsibilities include checking and monitoring the work of VNACs. They must hold the TDLB award D35 or V2.

Internal Verifier – A person who must hold the TDLB award D34 or V1, whose responsibilities include checking the portfolio and ensuring that assessments meet the national standards in a fair and consistent manner.

Level – A subdivision of the NVQ framework which is used to define progressive degrees of competence. The levels applicable to veterinary nursing are:

* *Level 2* – The person is required to perform a range of routine and non-routine activities within their work, with limited supervision.

* *Level 3* – The job role requires the performance of a wide

range of skilled and complex tasks, and also includes responsibility for the supervision of others.

NVQ – National Vocational Qualification, an award based upon occupational standards for the veterinary nursing sector upon which the veterinary nursing qualification is based in England, Wales and Northern Ireland.

Occupational Standards – These are the keys to the achievement of NVQs. They provide details of activities that veterinary nurses must be able to undertake competently in the veterinary practice. They are composed of elements made up of performance criteria, knowledge and understanding, and scope.

PC – Performance Criteria – The criteria that indicate the standard of performance required for the successful achievement of an element of competence.

QCA – Qualifications and Curriculum Authority – the accrediting body for NVQs in England, Wales and Northern Ireland. It is responsible for accrediting NVQs in all areas, and for auditing every awarding body to check that appropriate systems are in place and are being implemented effectively.

RCVS – Royal College of Veterinary Surgeons – the awarding body for the Veterinary Nursing NVQs.

Sector Skills Council – A body responsible for addressing the training needs of an industry and producing occupational standards. 'Lantra' is the Sector Skills Council for Veterinary Nursing.

SQA – Scottish Qualification Authority.

SVN – A student veterinary nurse, also known as a candidate when working towards the veterinary nursing NVQ.

TDLB – Training and Development Lead Body.

TP – Training Practice. A practice which fulfils the RCVS criteria to train veterinary nurses.

VNAC – Veterinary Nursing Approved Centre – a centre approved by the RCVS to provide veterinary nurse training and the necessary quality assurance of training and assessment.

This list is not exhaustive, and further information is available in Appendices A and B at the back of this book.

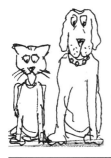

Chapter 1
Portfolio annexes

The portfolio annexes contain your vital training details, which may need to be assessed by the RCVS at any time. They will certainly need to be checked regularly by your assessor and internal verifier (IV). They must also be presented completed to date each time your IV checks your portfolio or it is submitted to the VNAC. Even at interim checks where only a small number of case logs are submitted, these details must also be presented.

As with the rest of the portfolio, you must always photocopy these forms to date before any submission. Also ensure that you actually present the original and not the copy.

Even though annexes E and F require joint compilation with your assessor, **all** of these forms are your responsibility and it is vitally important that they are updated regularly.

To ensure that you have spares it's a good idea to photocopy all of the sheets when you first receive your portfolio, along with copies of the log sheets. Or you may choose to download extra copies from the RCVS website.

Some of the actual master copies will continue through for both Level 2 and Level 3 (Annexes A and C), but all of the others will need to be new for Level 3.

Annex A

This covers your personal details, including your RCVS enrolment number and date and your full name and home address. Complete immediately upon receipt.

Annex B

This is the only section that may be easier for you to complete as you actually finish the Level 2 or Level 3 modules. However, it will be necessary for you to include a temporary contents page when submitting your portfolio for an interim IV check.

Every page of your portfolio must be numbered in the bottom right-hand corner, and obviously these must correspond with your contents page. It may be useful to create an individual module page numbering system eg MI – page 1, MI – page 2, M2 – page 5, M2 – page 6. This will make it easier to insert case logs without disrupting the whole numbering system. Similarly, appendices could be numbered eg a – 1, a –2, a – 3.

Annex Ci

This is your record of employment and practical training at a Training Practice (TP).

Again, your personal details should be entered as soon as you receive your portfolio, along with the name and address of your current TP.

Full or part-time training relates to your employment and not your college course.

Period of employment as an enrolled student – From is normally your RCVS enrolment date unless you have moved TP during your training. The *to* date is the date of submission for final verification. The rest of this table should also be completed on this day and duly checked and signed by your Practice Principal.

The following entry then includes the date following portfolio submission.

Annex Cii

Promptly record **any** absence from your TP, even including Bank Holidays, and ensure that your Practice Principal signs at the time.

The academic training record should be signed by your college course tutor, following each term or residential block.

Annex Ciii

This only needs to be completed and included in your portfolio if at any time during your training you change TP or VNAC.

It is vital that the RCVS, your VNAC and your college course provider are informed immediately of any change of circumstances. A copy of this completed form could be used to inform them. It is a valid 'hard copy' and much safer than a telephone message or word of mouth from your assessor.

Remember also that it is your responsibility to inform the 'big three' (RCVS, VNAC and your college!) of any change of personal details, such as name and home address.

If you forget to inform your VNAC it may mean that some of your logs are not internally verified – or worse still, they are no longer current.

The RCVS states that: 'Failure to notify a change of Centre or Training and Assessment Practice may result in loss of recordable training time'.

Annex D

This is an authentication of everyone whose signature appears in your portfolio.

Complete your own details and sign as indicated as soon as you receive your portfolio, but remember to ask all assessors and witnesses to sign this sheet at the same time as signing off a completed log sheet. This is to ensure validity and currency, but also acts as a safeguard just in case that particular person should leave the practice.

Your assessments will normally be carried out by your named assessor; however, it is fine to include witness statements from other personnel. This will normally be a vet or a qualified VN colleague, but occasionally your witness can be some other suitably experienced person, such as a receptionist, or even a client. Obviously the credibility of these witnesses will be checked by your IV, and your assessor will have signed off the log sheet on the strength of this and the witness testimony.

Try to let the prospective witness know in advance that you would like them to act as an evidence gatherer.

The witness statement should ideally be on your TP's headed notepaper, contain all of your details (name and enrolment number), and of course the date. It should just give a brief description of how competently you performed your role. Witness statements are evaluated by your assessor and taken into account as assessment evidence.

The witness may prefer to sign and comment on your case log instead of providing a witness statement. This must then, of course, be evaluated and countersigned by your qualified assessor.

Witness statements should be positioned in your portfolio after that particular case log. Do not include too many witness testimonies that refer to situations when your assessor was not present.

Annex E

There are separate tracking records for Level 2 (Ei) and Level 3 (Eii).

On receipt of your portfolio complete all of your usual personal details and the name of your qualified assessor.

Photocopy a number of these sheets and use one for your own personal tracking through your work. The original will be dated and initialled by your assessor as each case log is completed and signed off.

When the case logs are internally verified your IV will tick off and date each box in red ink. Occasionally the EV (External Verifier) will make spot check endorsements: they use green pens. So, don't ever be tempted to 'decorate' your portfolio with different colours: stick to black, or it could get confusing!

Annex F

Once again there are separate sheets for both levels.

Complete your usual details, then photocopy plenty of these planning sheets. Many will be needed because these will be updated by you and your assessor at your weekly planning tutorial session.

Planning assessments is a joint responsibility between the assessor and candidate. They will also use this form to identify your progress.

Always discuss with your assessor before working on a case for assessment. They can inform you of the suitability for that particular case in respect of variation, cross-referencing, standards, etc. This will most likely save you time! Use diaries, consultation appointments and theatre arrangements to help with your planning. Some TPs use separate notice boards to inform other members of the practice team of what you need to do, so that they are prepared to act as witnesses if your assessor is not around.

Your portfolio must be updated and reviewed regularly as part of training, and the RCVS recommends that this form reflects your weekly tutorial sessions. Obviously in a busy practice, and at times of illness or holidays, there will be many missed opportunities and situations where planned evidence gathering needs to be delayed. Your assessor will indicate any problems and rescheduling on the plan.

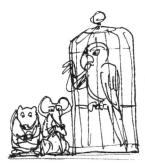

Chapter 2
Portfolio case log structure

Where and how should I start?

Assuming that the portfolio annexes have been entered, the next job is reading and beginning to make some sense of the occupational standards (see Chapter 4).

Do not attempt to read them all at once, but study each element as you begin the relevant portfolio module.

Appendices relevant to the module should be started (see Chapter 3).

Remember that you must always be guided by your assessor and follow your current assessment plan. However, you may find that one of the easiest modules to begin with is Module 5a Basic Animal Management.

I am not very confident of working on computer: Is it OK to handwrite the logs?

Yes. You can handwrite or print or wordprocess, whichever you feel the most comfortable with. However, it is possible that in the future the student will need to demonstrate information technology skills.

Handwriting must be neat and legible. Pencil is not allowed. Black ink is preferable because it actually photocopies much clearer than blue.

Can some logs be wordprocessed and some handwritten?

That would be fine. Most logs will actually be a combination of both, because even on a nearly perfect wordprocessed log there may need to be assessor questioning in order to complete and cover all of the standards.

Always back up and save wordprocessed work. You will also still need to photocopy every completed log because assessor comments and signatures must be handwritten, and this will be the only signed and truly authentic copy attributable to you.

If I do handwrite the case logs, I may not have enough space in some of the boxes

The size of the box is indicative of how much information to enter. Sometimes a great deal of information is unnecessary, and you may have covered some of it before. Common examples here may be convalescent feeding of high-energy clinical diets and their components, or the restraint of a dog for cephalic venepuncture. If common procedures have been described once then this is sufficient. Or you may choose to demonstrate your knowledge with a suitable appendix (see Chapter 3).

Where necessary, you may extend the box on the back of the sheet, or include an extra sheet. You will always need to set extra information out with appropriate headings, and extra page numbers must be entered on the contents pages.

Can I use bullet points for all of the logs?

Yes, for most. The exceptions would be Module 2c Detailed Client Information and the expanded case reports in Level 3 for Medical and Surgical Nursing. Also, the boxes that ask for your opinions and conclusion to a risk assessment require a detailed explanation, as of course do your reflective comments at the end of each log.

Bullet points are often easier to construct, tend to be clear and concise, but must still include descriptions where necessary. As you gain in confidence you may prefer to form paragraphs in later logs.

The expanded case reports are your chance to demonstrate detail and literacy.

Must I enter my name and RCVS enrolment number on every case log, appendix and even extra sheets of evidence? This seems to be a pointless repetition exercise

Each sheet in your portfolio is individual but contributes to your personal portfolio as complete authentic evidence of only your own work. Therefore, every sheet must be identifiable to you and must be signed and dated on completion.

You may decide to formulate a typical header on the computer for all additional sheets. This would contain all of the relevant boxes to ensure that you don't forget any important point, including your assessor's details, signature and date. It would be just as simple to transpose this on to a computer document as it would be to photocopy plenty of examples and to cut and paste as required. For example:

Student's name	VN enrolment no.
Student's signature	
Assessor's signature	Assessor's qualifications
Assessor's name	Date

Does every sheet of evidence have to be signed by my assessor?

You should present your case logs and any other relevant evidence to your assessor within a few days of the evidence occurring, or the assessment as agreed by your assessor. During a tutorial the assessor will highlight any points requiring correction and question you on your underpinning knowledge of the case and any other of the occupational standard PCs requiring extra evidence. Then, when your assessor is happy that you have demonstrated competence, they must sign and date each document.

In order to show currency of cases all of this authorisation must occur within a two-week period. Case logs that show a long interval between the evidence occurring and the assessor signatures cannot be submitted as current evidence. In exceptional circumstances the assessor can explain any time delay in the Assessor Comments box.

How should I describe the case number identification?

Keep this as clear and easy to classify as possible. Simplicity will help everyone involved, especially when cross-referencing cases. However, the case must relate to the actual patient record kept at your TP, so a computer or case reference number will need to be included.

Always remember client confidentiality and the relevance of the Data Protection Act.

The official reference could follow your simple identification, for example: 'Scamp – 5a.2 – Client reference 12345.'

A case reference is vital for your IV, who, on visits to your TP, is required to randomly check a small number of cases for authenticity against the actual client record.

What is meant by 'client type'?

The standards require you to have wide experience in dealing with different types of clients. These should include both new and current clients, because their specific requirements and practice protocols on dealing with clients will vary considerably.

Other modifications, such as 'difficult clients – aggressive, distressed', 'young and old' and disabilities should also be commented on at some point, or questions included by your assessor, but these do not necessarily need to be entered in the Client Type box. It can be really satisfying to describe how you assisted a client with special needs and can form the basis of a really interesting log, for example Log sheets 2b and 2c, depending on the special requirements of the client.

Do I need to enter all of the case log boxes?

Yes, even the Yes and No boxes. This may often seem repetitive, but is relevant to a particular case and vital evidence to cover the standards. This also applies to boxes that require the patient's weight or age. If there was a rare occurrence when a patient was not weighed immediately, then the reason why must be given in your Comments section. This situation may arise in Module 5b, Basic First Aid.

Can I use abbreviations?

Yes, they are acceptable provided that the first time you use an abbreviation you also include the full word and a brief description as necessary. For example: 'Tammy's CRT was > 2 secs'. (Her capillary refill time was greater than 2 seconds. This was abnormally increased because the normal value is usually less than 2 seconds. This indicated that she had a reduced blood flow because of the blood she had lost as a result of the Road Traffic Accident (RTA). I measured the CRT by applying pressure to the gum, releasing my finger, then assessing the time taken for the blanched area to return to normal.)

In future logs CRT details can now be abbreviated because you will already have met the standard required.

You may find it easier to use an appendix for abbreviations, but the first time you use an abbreviation you would need to make a reference to the appendix. Text containing many abbreviations can look untidy and often be quite difficult to interpret, especially for your IV reading the log.

What about veterinary terminology?

Use correct medical and veterinary vocabulary and phraseology wherever you can. This is not expected on your first few logs, but progression must be evident in later logs, and certainly by Level 3.

This is an excellent way of demonstrating your background knowledge, especially if initially you also include a short definition, and it may also help you work towards your external examination! For example: 'The budgie was exhibiting dyspnoea (difficulty in breathing)'.

How important is spelling and correct use of English grammar?

In the case of terminology it is vital to check your dictionary, as standard computer word checks are often not accurate when dealing with medical terms.

Spelling mistakes and grammatical errors will be highlighted and possibly commented on by your assessor. So that it is not necessary for you to repeatedly rewrite your first logs, you can just correct above the error or in the margin. It is expected that by Level 3 you will have progressed considerably, as with your veterinary knowledge and nursing experience.

It is not uncommon for students to have dyslexia, or just a problem expressing themselves on paper. You must inform your assessor if you are at all worried, as they are obliged to make allowances for this **without** being judgemental. You should also mention any problems to your college tutor, as they may even be able to arrange extra help as required. Any problems, even personal problems that may be delaying or affecting your work, may need to be reported on IV reports, but this will be to your advantage, and confidentiality must always be respected by all concerned.

What about mistakes? My assessor wants me to keep writing a log until it is perfect

Alterations actually help to demonstrate your progression because they show that you understand the error. For this reason, and although it may look neater, the use of correction fluid is **not allowed** anywhere in the portfolio. Mistakes must be attributable to you.

Ensure client confidentiality by using a black marker pen to obliterate their name and address. You may need to mark both sides of the sheet, as imprints often appear on the blank side.

Should I always refer to generic names of treatments and drugs?

Generic names are a priority throughout, but you should always try to include both generic and retail names, particularly in the case of Module 2b, in order to demonstrate your pharmaceutical knowledge.

In relation to calculations, how much working out do I need to show?

Equations and reckoning must always be shown, especially in Modules 2b and 5c at Level 2, and Modules 7, Medical Nursing, and 10a, Anaesthesia, at Level 3.

In the case of topical medicines or anthelminthics, where the dose is stated on the packet, then a calculation may not be appropriate. However, you should always include the dose rate for the patient in 'mg per kg body weight' and the strength of the medication.

Can I include extra evidence in the form of photographs, photocopies from books, drug company and data sheet information, or even practice leaflets?

Commercially produced leaflets will not enhance your evidence unless you clearly state the reason for inclusion and highlight the parts relevant to your assessment. Only include extra information if it can be directly attributable to you. This applies particularly to practice information sheets, and should be included only if you actually produced the sheet yourself and it has subsequently been signed and dated by your assessor.

Photographs taken by you are superb evidence to show your actual involvement with a case and to exhibit equipment and kennels (Modules 5a and 9d). However, they should never be used without a short reference or as a substitute for a description.

Include any extra evidence immediately following the particular log, and remember to add page numbers and adjust your contents sheets accordingly.

The hospitalisation sheet looks really untidy and is splattered with blood. Can I rewrite it to make it look more presentable?

Hospitalisation, consent and all monitoring forms included as evidence should be copies of the actual one used at the time. Your input should be highlighted. Remember to obliterate client details (but maintain your client reference) and include your enrolment number. As with all extra evidence sheets, your assessor must sign and date the sheet and it should be positioned in order immediately after the corresponding log.

I am unsure what to enter in the Student's Comments box

This is your reflection on the case. Think back on what exactly happened and ask yourself:

* What was my actual role?

* How did I deal with the client?

- ☙ Were there any special requirements for the client or the patient?

- ☙ Could I have done anything any better?

- ☙ If the outcome was successful, why?

- ☙ What have I learnt from this case for the future?

Comment on all of these and you will have greatly enhanced your evidence and possibly even been able to incorporate some of those elusive missing occupational standard PCs that you have not found a place for elsewhere.

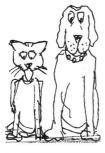

Chapter 3
Appendices

Appendices can be used wherever repetition is likely and to avoid duplicating information and save yourself some time. They are also an excellent way of demonstrating the depth of your knowledge.

Extra evidence can be included in a suitable amendment to an appendix, particularly if there isn't a relevant box in a log, yet the standards require you to include certain scope. You may also find this particularly useful if you have completed most of the logs for a particular module and then discover that there are a small number of PCs or scope missing. Of course these can always be covered by additional questioning by your assessor, but your own work will substantiate your evidence.

Many students use photos or even sketches to enhance their presentation and demonstrate authenticity.

Important points to remember:

* Ensure that each appendix contains all of 'the usual' extra evidence details, such as your name, RCVS enrolment number and signature, plus the signature of your assessor and of course the date of the signatures.

* Cross-reference carefully with all case logs, making sure that

you do include some detail in the log and refer to the particular appendix in question.

Reference the actual number/name of the appendix rather than just saying 'See appendix'.

If there is a great deal of information in one appendix then section it out under various headings and refer directly to one particular section only, in order to keep things simple. For example, if you have listed kennel sizes then you need to refer to which one was used and why.

❧ Number every appendix sheet and include the numbers on your contents pages. You may refer to page numbers as well as sections of appendices, but be careful not to overload your log sheet boxes with too much distracting evidence.

❧ All appendices should be included **together** at the front of your portfolio, just behind your RCVS annexes. This makes reference to them by your IV and assessor much easier than if they are mixed in with other log sheets. It also ensures that all of your evidence is together if your portfolio is handed in to your VNAC for an interim check. At this stage it is not vital to have included page numbers.

❧ When you begin to compile your appendices, if you refer to the occupational standards sections on *knowledge and understanding* these will help you to interpret what is required.

Table 3.1 illustrates how the knowledge and understanding sections of Element VN4.1 – Prepare accommodation for animals, can be incorporated into a commonly used appendix.

Table 3.1 Suggested appendix headings for Element VN4.1

Knowledge and understanding	Suggested headings	Suggested contents
(a) What type of accommodation is suitable for different animals and clinical conditions.	Kennel types, sizes and dimensions	Include all types used in your practice: Small, medium, large, glass fronted, walk-in kennels. Drawings, and photos are excellent to include here.
(b) Relevant regulations and guidelines.	The principles of health and safety regulations	Both of these sections should be covered by your Log sheet 1a. Therefore, another header is not necessarily needed here.
(c) and (d) Suitable environmental conditions, and the ways in which environmental conditions can be adjusted.	Environmental conditions	Explain the situation of the accommodation in the practice. List and give a brief explanation of: • lighting • heating • ventilation • humidity • noise. Explain how environmental conditions are adjusted for different species and clinical conditions.
(e) How to minimise stress.		This should be discussed on each log sheet in order to make it relevant to the case, species, treatment, handling, etc.

25

Table 3.1 *Continued*

Knowledge and understanding	Suggested headings	Suggested contents
(f) The types of bedding for different clinical conditions.	Bedding	Types of food and fluid should be relevant to each case. Types of bedding: Fleece bedding (including sizes), blankets, newspaper, straw/hay, bubble wrap, incontinence sheets. You may want to include a brief description of each, plus any merits or disadvantages. Cat litter and trays could also be included here.
(g) The security risks associated with animal accommodation.	Safety and security	• Cleanliness can be dealt with in 'cleaning' appendix, or in each particular log. • Security risks • Access. Give a brief description of how security is maintained. You may want to include: • The provision of double doors. • Window shutters/importance of checking/closing windows when dealing with cats and other species. • Types of catches on kennel doors and how to use them. • Authorised staff. • How and to whom problems are reported. You may choose to include isolation in this appendix, or perhaps in the cleaning appendix, or it may even warrant its own.

After discussion with your assessor it may be useful to decide which appendices you are going to do for each module. A good choice should both save you time and cover as many of the relevant standards as possible.

You can then begin these **before** attempting any logs and make amendments later as necessary (remember that any additions will need signing and dating).

In order to get you started, below is a list of 'suggested' appendices showing which units of the standards they cover. Included are headers and examples for the suggested content of each one.

Following this is a list of each module, with ideas of the appendices and headers for each, which could help you to complete each log sheet within that module.

Each appendix will ultimately be personal to you and must be individual to your TP, even though many background facts will be common to the syllabus.

Examples of suitable Appendices for Level 2

Appendix 1 (Level 2) – Animal accommodation

Units that can be covered: VN2.1, VN3.1, VN3.3, VN 4.1, 4.2, 4.3, VN6.1.

Refer to the example Appendix 1 above.

Appendix 2 (Level 2) – Health and safety legislation

Units that can be covered: ALL.

This appendix would cover virtually all areas of the standards for nearly all of the portfolio. Most of the occupational standards PCs require you to show evidence that you comply with health and safety regulations and guidelines at all times.

In addition, the knowledge requirements expect you to show an understanding of the principles and key points of the relevant health and safety regulations. Do remember, however, that you must still briefly explain the relevance and how each log relates to this appendix.

Health and safety is very important in a veterinary practice and it is vital that all staff be aware of their responsibilities for their own personal safety and that of their colleagues and visitors, and to follow all health and safety protocols and regulations.

The table, opposite, is an example which lists some of the various regulations and how they could apply to your TP.

Appendix 3 (Level 2) – Cleaning protocols

Units covered: VN1.2, VN1.4, VN2.1, VN3.1, VN3.2, VN4.1, VN4.3.

Here are some typical headings that you may want to include:

Cleaning products and dilutions

A table may be a good idea to show all of the cleaning products that you use regularly, for example:

Trade name	Generic name	Dilution/strength	Uses
		Give different examples appropriate to cases and situations	

Protective clothing

List examples, explain usage and disposal.

Health and Safety Legislation

Legislation	Relevant areas or work activities
The Health and Safety at Work Act 1974 and the Management of Health and Safety at Work Regulations, amended 1999	All areas
The Control of Substances Hazardous to Health 2002 (COSHH)	All areas, especially all aspects of cleaning, kennels, dispensary, consulting rooms, preparation room
The Ionising Radiation Regulations 1999	Radiography
Manual Handling Operations Regulations 1992	Lifting and transferring of patients and equipment. All areas, especially kennels and consulting rooms, handling and restraint
The Collection and Disposal Waste Regulations 1992	Disposal of waste
The Control of Pollution Act 1988	Anaesthesia, disposal of waste products
Environmental Protection Act 1992	Anaesthesia, disposal of waste, including radiographic processing chemicals
Reporting of Diseases and Dangerous Occurrences Regulations 1995	All areas – accidents can happen in all areas of practice
Display Screen Equipment Regulations 1992	Computer work and ultrasonography
The Medicines Act 1968, the Misuse of Drugs Act 1971 and the Misuse of Drugs Regulations 1985	All areas, especially dispensary and reception
The Electricity at Work Regulations 1989	All electrical equipment should be regularly checked and serviced
Fire Precautions Act 1971 and Amendment Regulations 1999	All areas

Signature	Student enrolment number	Date
Signature	Assessor	Date

Cleaning protocol for animal accommodation

Kennel routine

- Washing and drying of bedding – include contaminated items

- Feeding bowls and utensils

- Cat litter

- Infectious/contagious cases

- Precautions in case of zoonoses

- Special exotic requirements

- Care of patient during cleaning – show how the health and safety of the patient is maintained.

Cleaning protocol for examination rooms

- List basic procedures.

- Show how equipment and furniture should be positioned ready for use after cleaning.

- How would you identify damage or faults, and to whom would you report them?

Disposal of waste

Many students prefer to use a separate appendix here.

- Different categories and examples of types of waste.

- How each category should be disposed of – include the different types of clinical waste containers, storage until collection, and the protocol for collection.

Isolation

Again you may prefer to include more detail here and make it the subject of another appendix, or barrier nursing protocols can be included in one of your seven cases used in Module 5a – Basic Animal Management.

Appendix 4 (Level 2) – Methods of payment

Can cover almost all of Element VN1.3 and VN5.1, VN5.4.

Suggested headings:

Who normally deals with payments

How and when? Are payments usually paid directly following consultation or visit, or on collection of an admitted patient?

Protocol for invoicing of clients

How are fees worked out and VAT included?

Protocol for cash payments

Protocol for payment by cheque

Protocol for card payments

Appendix 5 (Level 2) – Vital signs

Units that may be covered: VN2.1, VN2.2, VN2.3, VN3.2, VN3.3, VN4.2, VN5.3, VN6.1, VN6.3.

This is one of the most commonly used appendices and, along with Health and Safety, it will also apply to your Level 3 portfolio.

You may want to include the protocol for taking temperature, pulse and respiration. A short description of capillary refill time and/or mucous membrane colour could also be included. You will probably find that a table provides a useful format to show the variations of clinical parameters.

Examples of typical headings and contents:

Taking the temperature

- ❀ Type of thermometer
- ❀ Protocol
- ❀ Abnormalities and possible causes.

Assessment of respiration

Include abnormalities.

Taking the pulse

- ❀ Commonly used sites
- ❀ Protocol
- ❀ Abnormalities.

Normal ranges for different species

Species	Temperature (°C)	Pulse (beats/min)	Respiration (breaths/min)
Canine	38.3–38.7	60–180	15–30
Feline			
Cavy			
Other			

Suitable appendices that relate to Level 2 modules

Module 1 – Health and safety and personal performance

Appendices 1,2,3,4.

Module 2 – Reception and client support

Appendices 2, 3, 4.

Module 3 – Admit and discharge animals

Appendices 1, 2, 4, 5.

Module 4 – Prepare for and assist with medical veterinary procedures and investigations

Appendices 1, 2, 3.

Module 5 – Basic nursing

Appendices 1, 2, 3, 5.

Following are two very different types of case log. Both show suitable references to the appendices used above. Consequently, if sufficient detail were to be included in each relevant appendix then many of the standards applicable to each section would be adequately covered.

See Log sheet 4a

See Log sheet 5a

LOG SHEET 4a - PREPARE FOR AND ASSIST WITH MEDICAL PROCEDURES & INVESTIGATIONS

Student Veterinary Nurse's Name:		Lara Apso	VN Enrolment No:		F56417	
1. Case Details:	**Species:**	Rabbit	**Age:**	3 years	**Sex:**	Female
	Breed:	Dwarf Lop	**Weight:**	1.3 Kg		

2. Procedure prepared for:

3. Date: 14-2-04

Clipping and cleaning the rabbit's matted and dirty perineal area.

Assessor's Comments:

4. Preparation of the environment in which the procedure took place:

- I ensured that all of the windows and doors were closed in the prep area in order to make the room secure.
- I checked that all surfaces were clean and tidy and materials used previously had been put away in their proper place or disposed of correctly (Ref appendix 3, cleaning protocol for examination rooms and disposal of waste).

5. Preparation of the equipment and materials:

- Equipment prepared: clippers (size 10 blade), scissors, Chlorexhidine ('Hibiscrub'), water bowl containing warm water, surgical gloves for me and the Vet, cotton wool, paper towels, towel
  I checked the clippers to make sure they were in working order.

34

6. Assisting with the procedure: Describe the following briefly;

How the animal was prepared, handled and restrained;

- I gently lifted the rabbit from the cat carrier and placed him in normal sitting position on the table.
- I placed one hand over his back whilst the Vet examined the area.
- She was then gently rolled over into dorsal recumbancy and I placed my hands underneath to steady her whilst the vet clipped and cleaned the area.
- Following the procedure I placed her back into the cat carrier and attached a water bottle to the cage. She was collected by the owner 1 hour later.
- The table was cleaned and tidied and waste fur disposed of in the clinical waste bin.

State if any additional information was necessary in order to assist with the procedure, eg previous records, instructions manuals/reference materials;

- The rabbit's case record details were checked to be the same as the label on the cat carrier, before I removed her from the cage.
- Following the procedure, in accordance with the Vet's instructions I advised the owners about a product 'Rearguard' which can be used to prevent myiasis (fly strike) in rabbits. The patient was not infected on this occasion but during the summer it is likely that a dirty perineal area can attract flies to lay their eggs. I supplied the relevant leaflets to the clients.

Any other details about your role in assisting with the procedure and monitoring of the animal;
Throughout the cleaning procedure I was continually observing the rabbit's heart rate and breathing patterns **(Ref Appendix 5 – normal ranges for rabbit)** to ensure that she was not distressed in any way.

Student's Comments and Signature:

Comments:

Restraint of rabbits is often quite difficult because if they struggle they can easily injure their back. This patient was well behaved but using this 'special' rabbit handling technique helped to relax her even more. By placing the rabbit in dorsal recumbancy with one hand cupping its back and the other supporting its head, it became very calm and almost mesmerised.

The evidence in this log sheet is a true account of the case/procedures described and my involvement therein. The work undertaken in compiling the log is my own.

Student veterinary nurse's signature ... *Lara Apoo* ....

Note – This is an example of a case log prior to evaluation, hence the absence of the Assessor Statement Box with the Assessor signature, qualifications and date.

LOG SHEET 5a - BASIC ANIMAL MANAGEMENT

Student Veterinary Nurse's Name:		Germaine Pointer	VN Enrolment No:		F2525
1. Case Details:	**Species:**	Feline	**Age:**	2 years	
	Breed:	Domestic Shorthaired	**Weight:**	3.4 Kg	
			Sex:		Male
					N

Assessor's Comments:

3. Reason for hospitalisation:

The patient was brought in for a veterinary consultation in the afternoon surgery. Earlier in the morning the owner had sprayed the cat with a proprietary flea spray from the supermarket and the cat seemed to have a reaction to the spray. The patient had been twitching and his eyes were exhibiting nystagmus (involuntary side to side movement of his eyeballs). He appeared to be partly conscious and reacted to us calling his name.

The patient was admitted for observation and treatment as necessary.

4. Type of accommodation and bedding material used, to include: any relevant environmental factors

I prepared a small sized kennel (**Ref: Appendix 1 – Kennel sizes**) in order to allow space for him to move, by lining the kennel with newspaper and placing a Vetbed for warmth and comfort. An end kennel was prepared because this is positioned away from the dogs and likely to be quieter.

I also placed a litter tray in the corner of the kennel.

Bagpuss's body was covered by a light blanket.

The consent for treatment form and hospital records were attached to the kennel door and relevant details were recorded in order to inform all staff of the patients condition and the nursing care required.

5. Accommodation cleaning protocol, to include: type of disinfectant, dilution of, mechanical cleaning procedures, frequency of cleaning and disposal of waste:

The kennel was cleaned once daily with 'Trigene' (**Ref: Appendix 3 for dilution and cleaning protocol**) Cages are normally cleaned more frequently but in this case the Vet had instructed to keep disturbance to a minimum. So it was only cleaned when soiled. All soiled cat litter and newspaper was disposed of in the yellow clinical waste bin (**Ref: Appendix 3 – disposal of waste**). The Vet bed had been urinated on overnight so this was washed in the washing machine using non– biological washing powder then dried in the drier.

37

6. Feeding Regime:

No food was given on the first day , but once the shaking subsided and full consciousness was restored then a small bowl of water was offered but he did not appear to drink until the following morning.

On the second day he was bright and alert so half a can of Hills' a/d was given. (This is tasty and very concentrated due to the high fat content, so would provide him with the necessary calories for basic maintenance). This food was accepted readily so the other half was given 4 hours later.

A small bowl of water was put into the cage and the cat drank approx.20–30mls throughout the second day.

7. Nursing care and monitoring of the animal: Please give details of grooming, wound management, cleaning, monitoring of vital signs and "TLC".

Due to his condition on first admittance the cats kennel was kept partially covered in order to darken his environment and thus keep external stimulation to a minimum. Also for this reason his temperature was not checked regularly but I did observe his respiration patterns from outside the kennel. Rate was initially slightly increased but this and the depth returned to normal following his injection of Diazapam. (**Ref Appendix 5– Assessment of respiration, for normal feline respiration rate)**

Date(s) specify duration of hospitalisation ......01-02-04 to 03-02-04 ....

8.. Medication administered: (details can be cross referenced to Log 5c)

0.30ml of Diazepam was administered by the Vet shortly after admission. I restrained the cat for injection into the right jugular vein : Cross Ref: **5c Admed ' Bagpuss'**.

38

Student's comments, to include: the part the student has played in this case:

Comments:

This was an interesting case as the Vet was initially unsure whether it was the spray that had caused the fits.

As with any convulsions the animal should be observed whilst external stimulation must be kept to a minimum.

His recovery was uneventful following the sedative injection of Diazapam.

Copy of hospitalisation record attached   YES ☐   NO ☑

The evidence in this log sheet is a true account of the case/procedures described and my involvement therein. The work undertaken in compiling the log is my own.

Student veterinary nurse's signature   …Germaine Pointer…………………………………………………

Note – This is an example of a case log prior to evaluation, hence the absence of the Assessor Statement Box with the Assessor signature, qualifications and date.

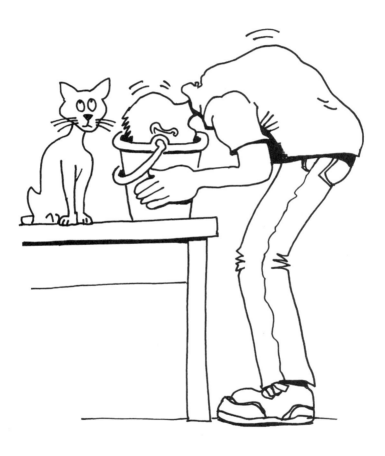

"A small bowl of water was offered but he did not appear to drink until the following morning."

Examples of suitable appendices for Level 3

Appendix 1 (Level 3) – Health and safety legislation

Units that could be covered: ALL.

As in Level 2 this appendix would cover virtually all areas of the standards for nearly all of the portfolio. Most of the occupational standard PCs require you to show evidence that you comply with health and safety regulations and guidelines at all times.

In addition, the knowledge requirements expect you to show an understanding of the principles and key points of the relevant health and safety regulations. An example of suitable legislation, showing how it may apply to your TP, is shown in the table overleaf. Do remember, however, that you must still briefly explain the relevance and how it relates to each log, in a similar way to the example table in Appendix 2 (Level 2) (page 29).

Appendix 2 (Level 3) – Infection control procedures

Units that could be covered: VN7, 8, 9, 10, 12, 13, CU2.

Most of these scopes, and consequently at least one of each relevant PC, will be able to be covered. Disposal of waste materials could be included in this appendix, which may then cover even more PCs. You may prefer to do a separate appendix just for disposal of waste. Details could include routine disinfectants/antiseptic solutions and dilutions.

Examples for headings

* Procedure for cleaning work surfaces.

* How different environmental conditions may affect infection control, eg appropriate ventilation.

* How direct/indirect contact with other animals is minimised or controlled.

🐾 How potential dangers, such as injury or zoonoses are minimised.

🐾 Disposal of waste.

Health and safety legislation

Legislation	Relevant areas or work activities
The Health and Safety at Work Act 1974 and Management of Health and Safety at Work Regulations, amended 1999	All areas
The Control of Substances Hazardous to Health 2002 (COSHH)	All areas, especially laboratory, handling of drugs, radiography, including dark room, anaesthesia, cleaning and sterilisation
The Ionising Radiation Regulations 1999	Radiography
Manual Handling Operations Regulations 1992	All areas, especially anaesthesia and surgical nursing
The Collection and Disposal Waste Regulations 1992	Disposal of waste
The Control of Pollution Act 1988	Anaesthesia, disposal of waste products
Environmental Protection Act 1992	Anaesthesia, disposal of waste
Reporting of Diseases and Dangerous Occurrences Regulations 1995	All areas: accidents can happen in all areas of practice
Display Screen Equipment Regulations 1992	Computer work and ultrasonography

Signature	Student enrolment number	Date
Signature	Assessor	Date

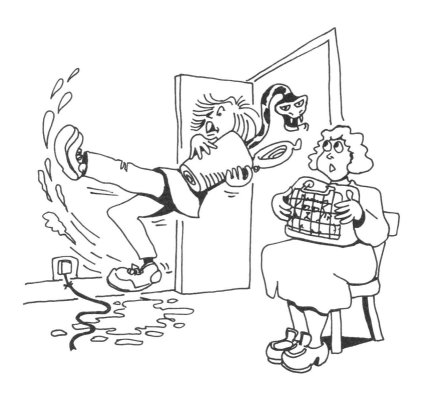

Ignore Health and Safety issues at your peril!

Appendix 3 (Level 3) – Environmental conditions and adjustment for different species

Units that could be covered: VN7.2, VN9.2, VN10.1, 10.3, VN11.3, VN12.2, 12.4.

This appendix may be a little limited because it will only be able to cover basic hospitalisation requirements (similar to your accommodation appendix in Level 2), and each case will most likely require more specific detail, depending on the species in question.

Appendix 4 (Level 3) – Normal clinical parameters and vital signs

Most units can be covered.

You will probably have included this at Level 2, but it is still very relevant for most Level 3 modules.

Include normal ranges for all species covered in your logs.

Appendix 5 (Level 3) – Confirmation of the animal's condition

Units that may be covered: VN7.1, 7.2, 7.4, VN8.1, 8.2, 8.3, VN9.1, 9.2, 9.3, VN10.2, 10.3, VN12.1, 12.2.

Each log will require a special reference which relates to the procedure to be performed and the log and module in question.

This appendix could include how you:

* Confirm the patient's condition by using available information, such as computer records, consent forms, hospitalisation sheets, kennel numbers

* Communicate the information to the veterinary surgeon

* Use special procedures, such as individual patient

identification – eg collar labels
* Use appointment books, procedure lists, etc.

Appendix 6 (Level 3) – Preparation of the patient for venepuncture

Units that could be covered: VN7.2, 7.3, VN8.1, 8.2, 8.3, VN9.1, 9.2, VN10.2, 10.3, VN12.1, 12.2, 12.3, 12.4.

This is not actually mentioned directly in the Level 3 standards, however, you may find that inclusion will save you a great deal of time and repetition when compiling many of the log sheets.

Include:

* restraint and positioning

* a description of the anatomy for commonly used veins

* basic equipment

* aseptic preparation

* the procedure

Appendix 7 (Level 3) – X-ray processing:

Units VN9.1, 9.3.

Suitable headings

* the processing unit

* preparation and maintenance/cleaning of the processor and solutions

* processing procedure

* possible problems

* advantages compared to manual processing techniques.

Appendix 8 (Level 3) – Appraisal of the Radiograph

Units VN9.3.

These details need to be entered in Box 11 of the case logs in Module 8a. However, good practice and health and safety legislation require us to produce a *satisfactory* and 'near perfect' radiograph of diagnostic quality. This appendix could therefore include *unsatisfactory* results that hopefully will never occur, such as:

- positioning errors
- processing faults
- exposure faults
- equipment faults.

Appendix 9 (Level 3) – The X-ray machine

Units VN9.1, 9.3.

- Short details about the machine type.
- Preparation, including use of light beam diaphragm.
- When radiography is finished.

Appendix 10 (Level 3) – Pre-operative preparation of the surgical site

Unit VN10.3

- Equipment, including clippers and antiseptic solutions.
- Procedure.

.

Appendix 11 (Level 3) – Preparation of the surgical team

Unit VN11.1.

- ❧ Antiseptics.
- ❧ Scrub technique.
- ❧ Donning of surgical clothing, including gloving.

Appendix 12 (Level 3) – Standard surgical kits

Units VN10.2, VN11.1, 11.2.

- ❧ Lists of basic packs.
- ❧ Suture needles.
- ❧ Suture materials.
- ❧ Instrument cleaning.

Note that sterilisation will be included in Log 9bi.

Appendix 13 (Level 3) – Procedure for disconnection of the patient from the anaesthetic equipment

Unit VN12.4.

Appendices as they relate to Level 3 modules

Module 6 – Laboratory and diagnostic aids

Appendices 1, 2, 3, 5, 6.

Module 7 – Medical nursing and fluid therapy

Appendices 1, 2, 3, 4, 5, 6.

Module 8 – Diagnostic imaging

Appendices 1, 2, 3, 5, 6.

You may also want to include extra evidence which is required for The scope and occupational standards PCs of VN9.3.

Module 9 – Surgical nursing and theatre practice

Most common appendices will apply here.

Section 9c – General Nursing requires six cases and two expanded surgical reports, so the following examples of Appendices 10, 11 and 12 may also be useful; however, these particular examples could be referred to in either of the expanded case reports and then used as a cross-reference for the other five cases. As always, discuss this idea with your assessor, because cross-referencing does require you to have used quite a large amount of detail on your first expanded report in order for this idea to be beneficial. Also, of course, progression still needs to be demonstrated throughout your portfolio.

Module 10 – Anaesthesia

Appendices possible: 1, 2, 3, 4, 5, 6, 10, 13.

Module 11 – Manage the availability of veterinary resources

Appendices 1, 2.

Included next is an example of a General Surgical Nursing log sheet case study with highlights to show how the relevant appendices can be referenced.

This is a very detailed log, which adequately covers many standards and scopes for VN10. This is typical of the standard of log that would be completed towards the end of your portfolio.

See Log sheet 9c

LOG SHEET 9c - SURGICAL NURSING – GENERAL

Student Veterinary Nurse's name:		Iris Setter	VN Enrolment No:	AN 073012	
1. Case Details:	**Species:**	Canine	**Age:**	5 years	**Sex:** Male(N)
	Breed:	Irish Setter	**Weight:**	24.4Kg	
2. Case No. Identification:		9C 3 Setter (computer ref. AL 123 'Red')	**Assessor's Comments:**		

3. Surgical procedure:

General anaesthetic – debride and suture wound on left ear pinna

4. Preparation of instruments, surgical equipment and materials:

I checked 'Red's' computer record and consulted the veterinary surgeon as to whether any specific surgical equipment or materials would be needed, in order that they could be prepared in advance. (**Ref. Appendix 5**)

I checked that the autoclave had adequately sterilised the necessary instruments (**Ref. Appendix 12 – List of basic packs – small kit**) by confirming that the Bowie-Dick indicator tape sealing the pack had changed to dark brown. I also checked all of the seals were intact and that there were no visible holes in the nylon film, and that the expiry dates on the pack were up to date. On opening the sterile packs I also checked that the chemical indicator strip within had changed colour (see Log 9bi).

The following presterilised equipment was positioned (having first been checked for damage or deterioration) ready for use, on the side bench in theatre:

- A pack of 10 additional swabs
- Surgical gloves (size 8)
- A range of suture materials, including monofilament polyamide - as instructed by the vet
- Scalpel blade – size 15
- Theatre attire, including face masks and caps.

Chlorhexidine (Hibiscrub) 1:20 , surgical spirit and cotton wool (**Ref Appendix 10 – Equipment**) – in this instance the eqiupment was placed on a trolley next to the table, where it could easily be reached and was less likely to be knocked over.

The clippers were fitted with a size 40 blade, checked for damage, and prepared for use (see Log 9d). They were positioned ready for use on the wall hook in the prep room.

Bandaging equipment was set out, including: sterile dressing ('Rondopad'), cotton wool, 7.5 cm padding bandage, 7.5 cm conforming bandage, and 7.5cm cohesive bandage.

The ambient theatre temperature was checked to be at 20°C, and the air conditioning was switched on.

Scrub suits and anti–static footwear were put on before entering the theatre.

5. Preparation of the animal for surgery:

'Red' was starved of food and water from 10.00pm the night before the procedure, and water was withheld from 8.00am on the morning of the operation. On admittance, at 8.30am, a consent form was completed. I confirmed the patient's details and procedure with the owner and also checked the computer details for any relevant history (**Ref. Appendix 5**) The dog was then weighed and placed in a prepared hospital kennel.

As the patient was less than 10 years old and there were no clinical signs to indicate that a blood test was necessary, pre–operative blood tests were not performed.

During the initial veterinary consultation the previous evening, 'Red' had received by subcutaneous injection; 1.5 ml (75mg) Carprofen ('Rimadyl') and 1ml (175mg) Amoxycillin ('Synulox'). These were given to provide pain relief and antibiosis respectively.

Prior to the procedure the Vet examined the patient and then administered the premed. Consisting of. 1.15ml (0.3mg) Acepromazine ('ACP') and 1.15ml (1.5mg) Butorphanol ('Torbugesic').

After approx. 20 minutes when an appropriate level of sedation had occurred, I restrained 'Red' for venepuncture into his right cephalic vein (**Ref. Appendix 6– restraint and vein preparation**)

The anaesthesia was then induced by the vet and maintained by another nurse.

The dog was positioned in left lateral recumbancy and a thick pad of cotton wool was placed in the external ear canal to protect the ear during surgical preparation. The right ear pinna was then clipped and prepared (**Ref. Appendix 10).**

He was then transferred via trolley to theatre and fitted with monitoring aids; pulse oximeter and oesophageal stethoscope and a final preparation of the site was completed as in (**Appendix 10 – immediately before draping).** Finally I directed the theatre lamp over the surgical field.

6. Assisting during the surgical procedure:

I assisted by:

- Helping the vet to prepare (**Ref**– Appendix 11– **donning of surgical clothing and gloves**).

- Opening and aseptically presenting to the Vet the previously autoclaved packet containing a fenestrated surgical drape) and the pack of swabs.

- Aseptically opening a small pack (**Ref** – **Appendix 12**) of previously autoclaved instruments and placing on the draped trolley.

- Aseptically opening and presenting (as in case log 9c.1 Westie) to the Vet, the scalpal blade and suture materials as and when requested.

- Counting all surgical materials during and after surgery.

- Disposing of waste as appropriate (**Ref-Appendix 2 – disposal of waste**). Used swabs were placed into the clinical waste bin.

7. Recovery from surgery (post-operative care):

I removed the drapes and monitoring equipment but anaesthesia was continued until the dressing was applied.

I bathed the sutured area and cleaned the surrounding bloody coat around his head using Chlorohexidine Gluconate ('Hibiscrub') –dilution 0.05%. I used separate swabs to avoid contamination of the wound then carefully dried the area using dry paper towels. I removed the cotton wool pad and checked the external his external ear canal for discharge or contamination from the wound. The wound was covered with the sterile dressing and I then reflected the injured left ear upwards. I placed a pad of cotton wool on top of the dog's head and folded the ear onto the pad. Then I applied another pad of cotton wool over the ear. This would protect the injured flap and help to absorb and control any post operative haemorrhage. Starting at the top of the head I applied the padding bandage around the head in a figure of eight pattern, leaving the opposite ear out of the bandage. Conforming bandage and finally cohesive bandages were also applied around the head in a figure eight pattern. Finally I indicated with a marker pen on the head, the direction of the bandaged ear. This would hopefully prevent accidental damage when removing the dressing at a later date.

In order to check that the dressing had not been applied too tightly I put 2 fingers underneath the dressing at the ventral aspect and both the rostral and caudal ends of the bandage.

For recovery, 'Red' was placed in lateral recumbancy, on a thick layer of 'Vet-bed', in the recovery room which is warm and secure. I continually monitored his breathing patterns and mucous membrane colour in order to ensure that the dressing was not interfering with normal respiration. They remained normal throughout (**Ref –Appendix 4 Assessment of respiration**). His ET tube was not removed until his gagging reflex had definitely returned (**Ref– Appendix 13– Removal of ET tube**). I continued to closely observe his breathing and other vital signs until he began to sit up when I then returned him to his hospital kennel. He was then observed for signs of haemorrhage, pain or shock but his parameters remained normal (**Ref: Appendix 4**). Interference with his dressing, head pressing or vocalisation may have indicted pain. If any problems had been observed then I would have reported directly to the Vet.

When 'Red' was beginning to attempt to stand, I telephoned the client to report on his progress and arrange a collection time for early evening. At collection instructions were given to the client on general post operative feeding and advise regarding the bandage. This was reiterated by giving out written instructions and a follow up appointment was made for 3 days time. The client was assured that she should contact us if any problems arose.

The operating theatre was cleaned and disinfected following the procedure as in (Log sheet 9a) and the consent form and anaesthetic record were filed in the lockable, secure metal filing cabinet in the office.

Date(s) to include full timescale range if appropriate. …….15-03-04 ………………………

Student's Comments and Signature:

Comments:

Following application of ear dressings it is vital that the patient is constantly monitored until recovery from the anaesthetic. I did not remove his ET tube until I was absolutely certain that there was no obstruction to his trachea from the dressing.

I am pleased that there were no post operative complications and the dressing stayed secure until his post operative check 3 days later when the Vet removed the dressing to reveal that the sutured pinna was uncontaminated and beginning to heal.

I advised the owner that 'Red' should continue to wear his buster collar for another 14 days, but his sutures could be removed 10 days following the surgery providing that there was total healing.

The evidence in this log sheet is a true account of the case/procedures described and of my involvement therein. The work undertaken in compiling the log is my own.

Student Veterinary Nurse's Signature... *Iris Setter*............................

Note – This is an example of a case log prior to evaluation, hence the absence of the Assessor Statement Box with the Assessor signature, qualifications and date.

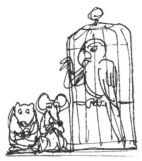

Chapter 4

National occupational standards

Discussions with both student veterinary nurses and assessors during practice visits, college course tutorials and assessor workshops have made it abundantly clear that the most difficult and perplexing aspect of portfolio compilation is the relationship between the case logs and the national occupational standards.

The aim of this chapter is to:

🐾 put this relationship into context

🐾 explain how an understanding of the relationship between the case logs and occupational standards can enhance the production of a comprehensive portfolio that satisfies all the criteria of the occupational standards.

🐾 avoid unnecessary repetition of evidence presentation, which will be reflected in a reduced workload for both student and assessor. The chapter is written from the student's perspective of these concepts; a later chapter covers the assessor's perspective.

What are the national occupational standards?

The national occupational standards are pivotal to the NVQs, forming the basis of all assessment. They provide details of the activities that a student veterinary nurse should be able to undertake to demonstrate competence in veterinary nursing skills. There are currently two levels of Veterinary Nursing NVQ standard, Levels 2 and 3, Level 3 being the highest. The standards were written by the Sector Skills Council (Lantra).

The standards comprise a number of components:

Units

Grouping of activities carried out in the workplace, all of which are mandatory

Elements

Describe the activity or outcomes that the SVN should be able to demonstrate to prove their competence in that unit

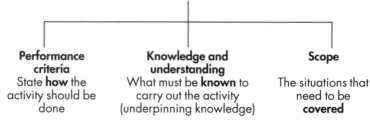

Performance criteria	Knowledge and understanding	Scope
State **how** the activity should be done	What must be **known** to carry out the activity (underpinning knowledge)	The situations that need to be **covered**

All aspects of the standards must be achieved to prove competence.

If we consider the Level 2 standards there are eight mandatory units that must be achieved:

☙ Unit CU2 – Monitor and maintain health and safety

☙ Unit CU5 – Develop personal performance and maintain working relationships

☙ Unit VN1 – Carry out veterinary reception duties

☙ Unit VN2 – Prepare for and assist with medical procedures and investigations

☙ Unit VN 3 – Provide nursing care to animals

☙ Unit VN4 – Care for animals in accommodation

☙ UnitVN5 – Support clients in caring for animals

☙ Unit VN6 – Admit and discharge animals.

If we focus on Unit VN6 – Admit and discharge animals, it can be seen that it is composed of three elements:

☙ VN6.1 – Admit animals for care

☙ VN6.2 – Communicate with clients regarding the progress of inpatients

☙ VN6.3 – Discharge animals from care.

It can be seen from Table 4.1 that Unit 6.1 – Admit animals for care is composed of:

☙ Performance criteria 1–10.

☙ Knowledge and understanding a–f

☙ Scope A–C.

Table 4.1 Admit animals for care

Performance criteria – You must:
1. check the details of the owner and the *animal* for which admission is required
2. make the *animal's* records available at the time of admission
3. confirm the *procedure* for which the *animal* is to be admitted from its records and with the owner
4. check the owner understands what is to be done and why
5. consult a veterinary nurse or veterinary surgeon if you or the owner are in any doubt
6. complete the admission form with the *details* required in your veterinary practice
7. check the owner reads, understands and signs the consent form
8. inform the owner of how and when to establish contact with the practice to discuss the progress of the *animal* after admission
9. check the *animal* is safe and adequately restrained so the owner can leave it without risk of escape
10. maintain good health and safety practice when admitting animals

Knowledge and understanding – You must know and understand:
a   the importance of correctly identifying the client, the animal and the reason for admission
b   the reason for having the case record available and for completing a consent
c   the reason for the owner signing the form and why this must be informed consent
d   the procedure used in your practice for admitting animals and for maintaining contact with the owners while the animals are in hospital.
e   basic animal management, including handling and restraint
f   health and safety policy relating to animal handling and restraint

Scope – Admit the following *animals*:
A   (i)   cats, dogs and exotics *or*
     (ii) horses

Admit the following animals for the following *procedures*:
B   (i)   surgical
     (ii) medical

Record the following *details*:
C   (i)   client details
     (ii)   animal details
     (iii)   reason for hospitalisation
     (iv)   any relevant history
     (v)   any special care requirements
     (vi)   food and fluid intake
     (vii) weight

Note: Evidence from simulations is not acceptable for this element.

How do the standards relate to the portfolio and syllabus?

A simple overview of the relationship between the standards, the portfolio and the syllabus for both Level 2 and Level 3 is illustrated in Table 4.2.

Table 4.2

Level	Standards (Units)	Portfolio (Modules)	Syllabus (Sections)
2	VN 1–6 CU 2&5 (8 in total)	1–5	1–4
3	VN 7–13	6–11	5–12

Units denoted VN are specific to veterinary nursing; those denoted CU are common to other NVQs.

How can an understanding of the relationship between the standards and the case logs help in compiling the portfolio and furnishing evidence of competence?

The standards are the linchpin of portfolio compilation. An understanding of the relationship between the standards and the case logs will make satisfying the NVQ criteria much easier to accomplish.

The guidelines at the beginning of each module in the portfolio are a suggestion as to how you can satisfy the NVQ requirements, but they are **only** guidelines. The standards are what you must satisfy to prove your competence. They are your bible of portfolio compilation. This is a fact often misunderstood by both student and assessor. An appreciation of the Veterinary Nursing Occupational Standards and their routine use is essential for effective assessment.

The standards should be used to facilitate the planning and assessment of portfolio evidence. On each occasion you are assessed your competence will be matched against the standards

and recorded. This can be achieved by using your own copy of
the standards, which is provided by the RCVS to indicate the
competencies met in an ongoing manner, or alternatively using
some form of tracking chart.

As stated in the RCVS *Veterinary Nursing News* April 2004, *'It is
important to recognize that once an area of the standards has
been satisfactorily assessed, it need not be revisited'*. Stated
simply, if you can *satisfactorily demonstrate* your competence in
a module by completing fewer than the suggested number of case
logs indicated in the guidelines, this is acceptable. For instance,
in Module 10 Anaesthesia, 10a Anaesthesia records – 6 case
logs are given as a guide but if you can satisfactorily cover all the
relevant PCs and scope in less than this number, that is
acceptable. Remember, the performance criteria and scope only
need to be evidenced once. If the standards are used correctly as
described to assess performance, and cross-referencing is also
utilised, the number of case logs will be reduced, and
consequently the amount of time and effort needed on the part of
both student and assessor, which is by far the commonest criticism
levelled at Veterinary Nursing NVQ training.

Handy hints

* Familiarise yourself with the occupational standards.

* Do not expect to grasp an understanding of their use and
  relationship with the case logs overnight. It does take time
  and effort, but it is well worthwhile in the long run.

* Make detailed notes about the case log before attempting to
  write it up.

* Most importantly, before writing it, study the relevant units of
  the occupational standards.

* Having done this, consider how you might write the log to
  demonstrate competence of as many of the performance
  criteria and scopes as possible. Remember that Units CU2
  (Monitor and Maintain Health and Safety) and CU5

(Maintain Effective Working Relationships) features in most Level 2 modules.

* As you satisfy performance criteria and scope, tick them off on your copy of the occupational standards.

* Remember, you only have to cover the performance criteria and scope once!

* Do not make extra work for yourself or your assessor. Reduce the pain and the strain for you both and get to grips with the standards – it is not as difficult as you think. Trust us!

In the following section you will find examples of both Level 2 and Level 3 case logs which will illustrate how, by using the occupational standards correctly, you can improve the coverage of both performance criteria and scope in your case logs, demonstrate your competence more effectively, and reduce your workload.

Included in each example is a log which is barely satisfactory, indicating the performance criteria and scope covered, and a far superior log of the same scenario but appreciating the use of the occupational standards.

Level 2

Example 1: Module 3 – Admit and discharge animals

3a Admit animals for veterinary treatment
Unit VN6.

Before studying these two case logs read again Table 4.2, which contains the relevant performance criteria and scopes.

These two examples cover the same admission, but the second is a much more comprehensive case log

See Log sheet 3a (2Ex.)

of the procedure as it utilises the performance criteria to provide much greater evidence of competence.

Example 1

LOG SHEET 3a – ADMIT ANIMALS FOR VETERINARY TREATMENT

Student Veterinary Nurse's Name:		Sheba Inu		VN Enrolment No:	F715682	
1. Case Details:	Species:	Canine		Age:	11 years	Sex:	Male
	Breed:	Boston Terrier		Weight:	8.4 kg	Client Type:	Current Elderly
2. Case Number – identification:		Admit 1 (Computer reference 58142) Toddy		Assessor's Comments:		

3. Reason for admission ie Procedures:

The patient was admitted to enable a blood sample to be taken for a full blood profile including biochemistry.

Performance Criteria and Scope covered.
VN 6.1
Scope A(i) (Dog)
B(ii)
C(iii)

4. Date & time animal admitted: ......7/4/04, 8 30 am ...   5. Date animal discharged: ...7/4/04......

6. Information given to client when admitted:

The client was informed that the blood tests would be performed that morning at the practice.

She was asked to ring at 1 00 pm to arrange a convenient time to collect Toddy and to discuss the blood test results with the veterinary surgeon.

The client was also informed that a small area of fur would be clipped off the underside (ventral aspect) of the dog's neck.

VN 6.1B

62

7. Action taken by student on admission of the animal:

I directed the client into the nurse's room, which provided a quiet and private environment.	VN 6.1 1, 2 & 3 Scope C(i) (ii) & (iii)
I checked the owner's and patient's details against the computer records and confirmed that Toddy was to be admitted for a blood sample to be taken.	
I asked the owner to read through the consent form and explained the information contained in Box 6.	VN 6.17
The owner seemed very anxious and confused about what to expect so I tried to reassure her.	
I took Toddy from her and led him through to the hospitalisation area, where I placed him in a medium-sized kennel (Ref Appendix 2 Kennel sizes and construction) with a piece of vet bed.	

Student's Comments and Signature:

Comments:

I felt I admitted the patient correctly and reassured the client who was quite elderly and worried about leaving Toddy.

The evidence in this log sheet is a true account of the case/procedures described and my involvement therein. The work undertaken in compiling the log is my own.

Student veterinary nurse's signature .... *Sheba Inu* ....

Example 2   LOG SHEET 3a - ADMIT ANIMALS FOR VETERINARY TREATMENT

Student Veterinary Nurse's Name:		Sheba Inu	VN Enrolment No:		F715682	
1. Case Details:	Species:	Canine	Age:		11 years	Sex:	Male
	Breed:	Boston Terrier	Weight:		8.4 kg	Client Type:	Current Elderly
2. Case Number – identification:		Admit 1 (Computer reference 58142) Toddy	Assessor's Comments:			

3. Reason for admission i.e. Procedures:

The patient record showed that Toddy had been seen the previous evening by the veterinary surgeon who was concerned that Toddy may have been suffering from renal failure. She arranged for a blood sample to be taken the following day to confirm the diagnosis. A full blood profile including biochemistry was to be performed.

Performance Criteria and Scope covered.
VN6.1
Scope A(i)(Dog)
B(ii)
C(iii) & (iv)

4. Date & time animal admitted: ......7/4/04 ...8.30am...   **5. Date animal discharged:** ..7/4/04...............

6. Information given to client when admitted:

The client was informed that the blood tests would be performed at the practice that morning.
She was asked to ring at 1 00pm to arrange a convenient time to collect Toddy and to discuss the results of the blood tests with the veterinary surgeon.
The client was also informed that a small area of fur would be clipped off the underside of the dog's neck (ventral aspect) to enable the blood sample to be taken.

VN 6.1B

7. Action taken by student on admission of the animal:	
I directed the client into the nurse's room which provided a quiet and private environment.	VN 6.1,1,2&3. Scope C(i), (ii) & (iii)
I checked the owner's and patient's details against the computer records, confirming with the owner that Toddy was to be admitted for a blood sample.	
I confirmed with the owner that Toddy had:	VN 6.1 Scope C(vi)
• been starved from 8 00pm the previous evening as this could affect the blood test results.	
• water available up until 7 30am that morning.	
• not shown any additional signs of illness since seeing the veterinary surgeon the previous evening.	
I then read through the consent form, which I had prepared earlier from the computer record, with the owner to confirm all the relevant details including a contact telephone number. I explained the procedure that was to be performed but the owner was very concerned about the procedure and its implications. I asked the veterinary surgeon to have a reassuring word with her so that she fully understood the procedure that was to be undertaken and the reason it was necessary. I also explained to her all the information listed in Box 6. She then signed the consent form.	VN 6.14 & 6
	VN 6.15
	VN 6.17
I placed a practice slip lead onto Toddy for added security in case he slipped his collar and escaped. I returned his lead to his owner.	VN 6.1 9 &10
The owner seemed quite distressed at leaving Toddy therefore I had to firmly, but gently, explain that Toddy would be fine in our care. This appeared to reassure her.	
Once she had left the nurse's room I ensured the door was properly closed then led Toddy to the hospitalisation area. I checked that all the doors and windows were closed then placed Toddy in an appropriately sized medium kennel (Ref Appendix 2 Kennel sizes and construction) with a piece of vet bed. I fastened the security catches on the kennel.	VN 6.1 9 &10
I completed Toddy's computer records to indicate that he had been admitted and I generated a hospitalisation sheet. The consent form and hospitalisation sheet were attached to the front of the kennel. His details were also entered on the ward board.	VN 6.1
I then weighed Toddy and monitored his temperature, pulse and respiration and his capillary refill time (CRT) and recorded them on the hospitalisation sheet. The TPR were all within the normal range . (See Appendix 4 TPR) and his mucous membranes were pink with a capillary refill time of less than 2 seconds.	Scope C(i), (ii), (iii), (vii)

Student's Comments and Signature:

Comments:

This was quite a challenging patient to admit as the owner was very anxious about leaving Toddy and I had to be very calm and reassuring with both the client and Toddy as he became quite apprehensive. I felt I managed to put the client's mind at rest and eventually she was quite confident about leaving Toddy in our care. Toddy also quickly calmed down after I stroked and spoke to him in a quiet, reassuring manner.

The evidence in this log sheet is a true account of the case/procedures described and my involvement therein. The work undertaken in compiling the log is my own.

Student veterinary nurse's signature .... *Sheba Inu* ....

Note – This is an example of a case log prior to evaluation, hence the absence of the Assessor Statement Box with the Assessor signature, qualifications and date.

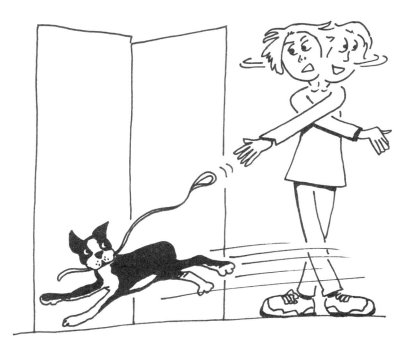

"I placed a practice slip lead onto Toddy for added security in case he slipped his collar and escaped."

Example 2: Module 2 – Reception and client support

2b Dispensing medication to clients
Unit VN 5.

See
Log sheet
2b (2 Ex.)

Now dust off the cobwebs from your occupational standards
and consult the relevant sections for the examples that follow.

Example 1

LOG SHEET 2b - DISPENSING MEDICATION TO CLIENTS

Student Veterinary Nurse's Name:		Jackie Russell	VN Enrolment No:		F19555	
1. Case Details:	**Species:**	Canine	**Age:**	3 years	**Sex:**	Male
	Breed:	Labrador	**Weight:**	37.25 kg		Neuter
2. Name of drug dispensed (include trade and generic names):			**Assessor Comments:**			
Drontal Plus – Febantel with praziquantel and pyrantel			*Performance criteria and scope covered*			
3. Legal dispensing category and drug classification:						
PML – Pharmacy and Merchants' List						
PML medicines may be supplied by a pharmacist or by a registered agricultural merchant or saddler.			*Scope VN5.4 A(i)*			
Veterinary surgeons may also supply them but only to animals under their care. This means that the animal must have been seen by the veterinary surgeon in the last 12 months.			*VN5.4 5*			
Oral (tablet) anthelmintic – wormer						
4. Dose given (include calculations):						
Dose:						
Data sheet recommends – 1 tablet per 10 kg body weight						
Dose given (include calculations):						
Dog weighs 37.25 kg						
Dose required = $\frac{37.25}{10}$ = 3.75 tablets. Dose given = 4 tablets						

5. Reason for administration and route:

Drontal Plus is a broad-spectrum oral wormer that can be administered at home by the owner. It is prescribed for the treatment of most canine roundworms and tapeworms common in this country. This includes the common roundworm *Toxocara canis* and tapeworms *Dipylidium caninum* and *Echinococcus granulosus.*

The tablets can be administered directly by mouth, crushed in food or hidden in a treat.

Scope VN5.3 B(i)
VN5.4 A(i)
VN5.4 4

6. Health & Safety, and other dispensing notes to include: 1) A duplicate copy of the dispensing label. 2) Health & Safety issues:

No eating, drinking or smoking whilst handling the tablet.

> FOR ANIMAL TREATMENT ONLY
> KEEP OUT OF REACH OF CHILDREN
> DRONTAL PLUS X4
> *Give 4 tablets as a single dose*
> 15-04-04
> Round and Tape Veterinary Surgeons,
> 2 Anthelmintic Way,
> Wormington-on-Sea

7. Additional advice/instructions given to client: (state how you ensured the client was able to administer the medication/treatment and any other information provided)

I reminded the client that they should worm their dog regularly every 3 months.
I gave them a proprietary leaflet which explains about *Toxocara canis.*

Date of dispensing: ...14–04–04...

Scope VN5.2 A(i)
VN5.2 2, 3, 4, 8

8. Briefly state the procedure carried out by you, when processing payments for the items dispensed (if applicable)

I added the cost of the tablets to the client record on the computer by selecting the automatic pricing option, and selecting the correct medication.
I informed the client of the cost and then processed a cash payment.

Scope VN1.3 A(i)
VN1.3 B(iv)
VN1.3 1, 2

Student's Comments and Signature:

Comments:

It's rewarding to inform owners about preventative health care for their animals.

The evidence in this log sheet is a true account of the case/procedures described and my involvement therein. The work undertaken in compiling the log is my own.

Student Veterinary Nurse's signature ....*Jackie Russell*..........

Note – This is an example of a case log prior to evaluation, hence the absence of the Assessor Statement Box with the Assessor signature, qualifications and date.

Example 2

LOG SHEET 2b – DISPENSING MEDICATION TO CLIENTS

Student Veterinary Nurse's Name:		Jackie Russell	VN Enrolment No:		F19555	
1. Case Details:	Species:	Canine	Age:	3 years	Sex:	Male
	Breed:	Labrador	Weight:	37.25 kg		Neuter

Assessor Comments:

2. Name of drug dispensed (include trade and generic names):

Drontal Plus – Febantel with praziquantel and pyrantel

Performance criteria and scope

covered

3. Legal dispensing category and drug classification:

PML – Pharmacy and Merchants' List

PML medicines may be supplied by a pharmacist or by a registered agricultural merchant or saddler.

Veterinary surgeons may also supply them but only to animals under their care. This means that the animal must have been seen by the veterinary surgeon in the last 12 months.

Scope VN5.4 A(i)

VN5.4 5

Anthelmintic – wormer

4. Dose given (include calculations):

Dose:

Each tablet contains – 50 mg praziquantel, 144 mg pyrantel and 150 mg febental

Data sheet recommends – 1 tablet per 10 kg body weight

VN 5.4 1, 4

Dose given (include calculations):

Dog weighs 37.25 kg

Dose required = $\frac{37.25}{10}$ = 3.75 tablets. Dose given = 4 tablets

VN 5.4 5

VN 5.2 3

It is difficult to administer 0.75 of a tablet. The vet directed that 4 tablets would be an appropriate dose for this dog as the data sheet says that 4 tablets are required for a dog weighing 35-40 kg.

5. Reason for administration and route:

Drontal Plus is a broad–spectrum oral wormer that can be administered at home by the owner. It is prescribed for the treatment of most canine roundworms and tapeworms common in this country. This includes the common roundworm *Toxocara canis* and tapeworms *Dipylidium caninum* and *Echinococcus granulosus*.

The tablets can be administered directly by mouth, crushed in food or hidden in a treat.

Scope VN5.3 B(i)

6. Health & Safety, and other dispensing notes to include: 1) A duplicate copy of the dispensing label. 2) Health & Safety issues:

The owner's attention should be drawn to the label especially re. 'Keep out of reach of children' and 'For animal treatment only'.

Hands should be washed after administering the medication.

No eating, drinking or smoking whilst handling the tablets.

Take care that the patient does not bite owner's fingers ring during administration by mouth.

Scope VN 5.3 C(i)

VN 5.3 8

VN5.4 6, 8

```
FOR ANIMAL TREATMENT ONLY
KEEP OUT OF REACH OF CHILDREN
DRONTAL PLUS X4
15–04–04
Give 4 tablets as a single dose
Round and Tape Veterinary Surgeons,
       2 Anthelmintic Way,
       Wormington-on-Sea
```

Scope VN5.1 A(i) B(ii)

7. Additional advice/instructions given to client: (state how you ensured the client was able to administer the medication/treatment and any other information provided)

These tablets had been dispensed previously, therefore I checked if the client was still happy to administer the 4 tablets at once.

Since this dog 'will eat anything', the client was happy to add the tablets to the dog's food.

I reminded the client that they should worm their dog regularly every 3 months, as a precaution to help prevent infestation. This client has two young children so I mentioned that the larval form of *Toxocara canis* can be dangerous, especially if ingested by children.

Regular worming of their own dog will reduce this risk.

I gave them a proprietary leaflet which explains about *Toxocara canis.*

I also informed the client that if they had any problems or queries then to give us a ring.

VN5.17

Scope VN5.2 A(i)

VN5.2 2, 3, 4, 6, 8, 9

Vn 5.3 4, 6

Date of dispensing: ...14–04–04...

8. Briefly state the procedure carried out by you, when processing payments for the items dispensed (if applicable)	Scope VN1.3 A(i)
	VN1.3 B(iv)
First I entered on the client's record the medication that had been dispensed and the advice that I had given to the client.	VN1.3 1, 2, 3, 4, 5, 6, 7, 8
I added the cost of the tablets to the client record on the computer by selecting the automatic pricing option, and selecting the correct medication.	
I informed the client of the cost and then processed a cash payment following the protocol shown in Appendix 4.	

Student's Comments and Signature:

Comments:

It's rewarding to inform owners about preventative health care for their animals. This client was particularly grateful that I also mentioned the importance of human welfare.   VN 5.2 4

Before dispensing the wormers I checked on the computer record that the client has been seen recently. This was just a routine wormer.   VN 5.4 1, 3, 5
As usual before dispensing any product, I also checked with the veterinary surgeon on duty that it was OK for me to dispense the tablets and advise the owner.

I noticed that the level of tablets in the dispensing box was quite low so I added another box to the drug order list. This is in accordance with our practice procedure. Twice weekly the head nurse checks this list when ordering from the wholesaler.   VN 5.4 2, 3, 7

The evidence in this log sheet is a true account of the case/procedures described and my involvement therein. The work undertaken in compiling the log is my own.

Student Veterinary Nurse's signature ...... *Jackie Russell*...............

Note – This is an example of a case log prior to evaluation, hence the absence of the Assessor Statement Box with the Assessor signature, qualifications and date.

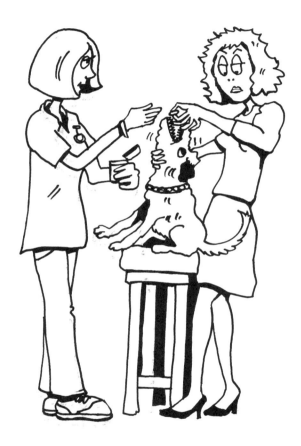

"Take care that the patient does not bite its owner's fingers during administration by mouth."

Level 3

The examples chosen to illustrate Level 3 are taken from two of the most difficult modules in the portfolio to cover all the scope of the standards in the log sheets alone.

Example 1: Module 8 – Radiography

8a Radiography
Unit VN 9.

There are three elements for this unit. Elements 9.1 and 9.2 relate to radiography whereas 9.3 is only concerned with ultrasound techniques and endoscopy.

Health and safety is a huge section in this unit, and most of it will be covered by the Health and Safety Risk Assessment; however, you should still mention health and safety in some form in each log, particularly where it is relevant.

The log sheets account for imperfections, but you may well not come across the scope requirements for VN 9.3 D normally in your choice of case log. Appendices could be useful to cover this, or your assessor can question you on any missing evidence.

Do not be tempted to include more than one view on one case log. It will be difficult to include all the necessary information, plus it increases the complexity of the log.

Remember, you must cover dogs, cats and exotics. **See Log sheet 8a (2 Ex.)**
Also, evidence from simulations is not acceptable.

Example 1

LOG SHEET 8a – RADIOGRAPHY

Student Veterinary Nurse's Name:		Bernard Saint				VN Enrolment No:		E 9876	
1. Case Details:	**Species:**	Canine				**Age:**	5 years	**Sex:**	Female Neuter
	Breed:	Jack Russell Terrier				**Weight:**	7.55 Kg		
2. Case No. Identification:		R 3 'Anna' (Comp Ref– April 141)	**Date image produced**		7th April 2004	**Assessor's Comments:**			

3. Area to be radiographed and reason:

Anna had been walking unsteadily on her hind legs for 3 days. Upon examination at consultation the veterinary surgeon suspected a problem of spinal origin. Anna was to be admitted for radiographs of her lumbar vertebrae.

Scope VN9.1 A(i) B(i)

4. Patient preparation, to include: means of restraint, eg manual, chemical (state medication used)

Food had been withheld from Anna since the previous evening to prepare her for the anaesthetic.
Anna was first premedicated with acepromazine (ACP) and butorphanol (Torbugesic).
General anaesthesia was induced by the vet 30 minutes later, using propofol (Rapinovet) intravenously. Anaesthesia was maintained via an endotracheal tube and T-piece circuit with halothane as the volatile agent.

Scope VN9.2 A(i) B(ii)

VN9.13

5. Recording equipment:	**Screen Type:**	Green rare earth (gadolinium oxysulphide). Rapid speed	**Film Type:**	Kodak green light sensitive 25 x 34 cm.	**Grid:**	Not used
6. Exposure Factors:	**FFD:**	75cm	**KV:**	70 kV	**mAs:**	7 mAs
7. View eg Ventrodorsal:	Lateral					

VN9.11

77

8. Positioning of animal, to include and positioning aids used:

Anna was then laid in left lateral recumbency with her lumbar vertebrae in the centre of the cassette.
Foam wedges were placed under Anna's mandible, cervical and lumbar spine to help ensure that her spine was parallel. Another foam wedge was placed under her sternum and further wedges between her legs to help prevent rotation of her body. Her forelimbs were drawn cranially and hindlimbs caudally and cords placed above the carpus and tarsus. These were secured to the table.

Scope VN9.1 C(iv)
VN9.1.3
VN9.2.2, 3

9. Centring details: state anatomical landmarks:

The primary beam was centred midway between the thoraco lumbar junction and the iliac crest and over the transverse spinous processes. This would be approximately over the fourth lumbar vertebrae.

VN9.2.3

10. Collimation of primary beam: state anatomical landmarks:

The beam was extended cranially to the 13th rib and caudally to the centre of the wing of the ilium. Dorsally the beam included the skin edges of the seven lumbar vertebrae and ventrally the beam included the dorsal third of Anna's abdomen.

VN9.2.3

11. Appraisal of radiographical quality to include: Comments/Action Taken: ✓ = Satisfactory   X = unsatisfactory

Positioning	✓	Collimation	✓	Centring	✓
Labelling	X	Contrast	✓	Density	✓

Scope VN9.3 A(i)
B(i), (ii), (iv)
C(i)

Comments and action taken if required:
The finished film had good contrast and was collimated to include only the area of interest.
A further film was taken to include all of the lumbar vertebra on a ventrodorsal view.
Unfortunately the X-rite tape and Left marker were not included in the film. I should have extended the dorsal collimation by approximately 5 cm in order to include these markers above the dog's body.

If artefacts were present, please state likely cause:
No artefacts were present.
The automatic processor's rollers are cleaned weekly in order to try to prevent any roller marks, and an old film is run through before commencing development in order to check function.

Scope VN9.1 D(ii) 9.3 D(iii) VN9.14

Please indicate how the radiograph was processed: (Please tick box) Manually ☐ OR Automatically ✓

12. Veterinary surgeon's diagnosis:

The veterinary surgeon could see no abnormalities, so it was decided that Anna should have complete rest for 1 week and the situation would be reassessed. If necessary a myelogram might then be undertaken.

Student's Comments & Signature:

Comments:
I was really pleased with the quality of this radiograph.

The evidence in this log sheet is a true account of the case/procedure described and my involvement therein.
The work undertaken in compiling the log is my own.

Student VN's Signature .... *Bernard Saint*...........

Note – This is an example of a case log prior to evaluation, hence the absence of the Assessor Statement Box with the Assessor signature, qualifications and date.

Example 2

LOG SHEET 8a – RADIOGRAPHY

Student Veterinary Nurse's Name:		Bernard Saint		VN Enrolment No:		E 9876	
1. Case Details:	Species:	Canine		Age:	5 years	Sex:	Female Neuter
	Breed:	Jack Russell Terrier		Weight:	7.55 Kg		
2. Case No. Identification:		R 3 'Anna' (Comp Ref– April 141)	Date image produced	7 April 2004			

3. Area to be radiographed and reason:

Anna had been walking unsteadily on her hind legs for 3 days. Upon examination at consultation the veterinary surgeon suspected a problem of spinal origin. Anna was to be admitted for radiographs of her lumbar vertebrae.
I confirmed with the veterinary surgeon the size of cassette to be used and the fact that a grid was not necessary.

4. Patient preparation, to include: means of restraint, eg manual, chemical (state medication used)

All available information (including Anna's computer record and consent form) was made available in order to confirm the procedure she was to undergo and the area to be viewed.

Food had been withheld from Anna since the previous evening to prepare her for the anaesthetic.

Anna was first pre-medicated with acepromazine (ACP) and butorphanol (Torbugesic). This was administered intramuscularly into the quadriceps muscle of the left hind leg on the instructions of the veterinary surgeon. She was held steady with her spine as straight as possible in order to minimise discomfort.

General anaesthesia was induced by the vet 30 minutes later, using propofol (Rapinovet) intravenously. Anaesthesia was maintained via an endotracheal tube and T–piece circuit with halothane as the volatile agent.

5. Recording equipment:	Screen Type:	Green rare earth (gadolinium oxysulphide). Rapid speed	Film Type:	Kodak green light sensitive 25 x 34 cm.	Grid:	Grid not required as area less than 10 cm thick
6. Exposure Factors:	FFD:	75cm	KV:	70kV	MAs:	7 mAs (20 mA x 0.35 seconds
7. View: e.g. Ventrodorsal:	Lateral					

Assessor's Comments:

Scope VN9.1 A(i)
  B(i)
  C(iii)
  D(i)

VN9.11,2

Scope VN9.2 A(i) B(ii) C(i)(ii)(iii)

VN9.11, VN9.21,5, VN9.33

VN9.13

8. Positioning of animal, to include and positioning aids used:

An X-rite tape label was prepared with the patient's name and date. Together with the LEFT marker they were placed within the primary beam collimation once the patient was in position. This must be done to enable identification of the radiograph and enable correct filing afterwards.

The cassette was lined up and collimated with the primary beam before Anna was then laid in left lateral recumbency with her lumbar vertebrae in the centre of the cassette. Great care was taken here during moving Anna in order not to exacerbate her condition in case there was a spinal fracture or disc dislocation.

Foam wedges were used to prevent the natural sagging and rotating of the spine and to ensure that it formed a straight line parallel to the cassette. Foam wedges were placed under Anna's mandible, cervical and lumbar spine to help ensure that her spine was parallel. Another foam wedge was placed under her sternum and between her legs to help prevent rotation of her body.

Her forelimbs were drawn cranially and hindlimbs caudally by cords placed above the carpus and tarsus. These were secured to the cleats on the table using a safe quick release figure-of-eight tie.

Throughout the positioning, Anna's vital signs were checked (REF Appendix ---) in order to detect any potential difficulties.

VN9.13

Scope VN9.1 C(iv)
VN9.2 2, 3, 4, 7

VN9.24

9. Centring details - state anatomical landmarks:

The primary beam was centred midway between the thoraco lumbar junction and the iliac crest and over the transverse spinous processes. This would be approximately over the fourth lumbar vertebrae; however the muscle masses around the vertebrae make it difficult to determine and palpate precisely the anatomical position of each vertebra.

VN9.2.3

10. Collimation of primary beam - state anatomical landmarks:

The beam was collimated by altering the dials which control the light beam diaphragm and turning on the light in order to identify the centre and borders of collimation.

The beam was extended cranially to the 13th rib and caudally to the centre of the wing of the ilium. Dorsally the beam included the skin edges of the seven lumbar vertebrae and ventrally the beam included the dorsal third of Anna's abdomen.

Once the veterinary surgeon was satisfied with the positioning we both moved behind the lead screen and I pressed the exposure button.

Scope 9.1 C(i)

VN9.23

81

11. Appraisal of radiographical quality to include: Comments/Action Taken: ✓ = Satisfactory   X = unsatisfactory

Positioning	✓	Collimation	✓	Centring	✓
Labelling	X	Contrast	✓	Density	✓

Scope VN9.3 D(i)

Comments and action taken if required:

The finished film had good contrast and was collimated to include only the area of interest, although to prevent the divergence of the primary beam from producing inaccurate images towards the edge of the collimation it is actually best to only include three or four vertebrae in each exposure. This greatly increases the number of exposures required so in order to reduce the cost for the client the veterinary surgeon decided in this instance to include all of the lumbar vertebrae in this one film.

VN9.3,1, 2

A further film was taken to include all of the lumbar vertebra on a ventrodorsal view.

Unfortunately the X–rite tape and Left marker were not included in the film. I should have extended the dorsal collimation by approximately 5 cm in order to include these markers above the dog's body. To remedy this I filled in a sticky label with all of the relevant details and attached this to the top right–hand side of the radiograph as soon as processing was complete.

VN9.14
VN9.38

If artefacts were present, please state likely cause:

No artefacts were present.

The automatic processor's rollers are cleaned weekly in order to try to prevent any roller marks, and an old film is run through before commencing development in order to check function.

Scope VN9.1 D(ii)
9.3 D(iii)
VN9.14, VN9.36

Please indicate how the radiograph was processed: (Please tick box)	Manually	☐	OR	Automatically	✓

12. Veterinary surgeon's diagnosis:

The veterinary surgeon could see no abnormalities, so it was decided that Anna should have complete rest for 1 week and the situation would be reassessed. If necessary a myelogram might then be undertaken

Comments:

I was really pleased with the quality of this radiograph. The positioning and processing were good.

Following the procedure and once the veterinary surgeon was happy with the diagnosis I turned off the X-ray machine and disconnected it from the mains, according to the local rules.

I filed both labelled radiographs in alphabetical order in the X-ray filing cabinet.

The exposure was recorded in the exposure book. I recorded the owner and patient details, including the patient's weight, the area that was radiographed and the setting used. I also commented on the fact that it was a good exposure. This record could then be used in the future to ensure accuracy when deciding on settings and so reduce the possibility of needing a repeat exposure, an essential requirement for health and safety.

The X-ray table and outside of the cassette was cleaned with Trigene (1:100 dilution) in order to prevent any cross-contamination or possible infection between this and the next patient.

VN9.3.4, 9.3.8, 9.3.6, 9.3.9, 9.3.11, VN9.3.15

Scope VN9.1 E(i), (ii)

The evidence in this log sheet is a true account of the case/procedure described and my involvement therein.
The work undertaken in compiling the log is my own.

Student VN's Signature ...... *Bernard Saint*..............

Note – This is an example of a case log prior to evaluation, hence the absence of the Assessor Statement Box with the Assessor signature, qualifications and date.

Example 2: Module 6 – Laboratory and diagnostic aids

6a Laboratory and diagnostic aids (6ai Packed cell volume) VN 7.

This unit is composed of four elements. Again, all the performance criteria and scopes are difficult to cover in the case logs alone and additional assessor questioning or extra reports may be necessary to prove your competence. Simulations are not acceptable for this module.

Obviously not all the performance criteria and scopes can be covered in one log, but with a better understanding of the relationship between case log compilation and the occupational standards the construction and development of your portfolio will be vastly improved.

See
Log sheet
6a (2 Ex.)

Example 1

LOG SHEET 6a - LABORATORY & DIAGNOSTIC AIDS

Student Veterinary Nurse's Name:		Ben Gall	VN Enrolment No:		F62195	
1. Case Details:	Species:	Feline	Age:	3 yrs 5 mths	Sex:	Male
	Breed:	Domestic Shorthair	Weight:	4.8 kg		

2. Case No. Identification: Lab 6a1 (Computer reference 44192) Basil

Assessor's Comments:

Performance criteria and scope covered.

3. Type of procedure and reason for test:

A packed cell volume (PCV) was performed to investigate if the patient was anaemic.

VN7.1 Scope A(i) (Cat)
B(i) (Blood)

4. Preparation of animal and pre-test procedures:

I clipped a small area of fur from the ventral aspect of the cat's neck over the left jugular vein. The area was then cleaned with a chlorhexidine (Hibiscrub) 1:20 solution and swabbed with spirit to prevent introduction of infection and contamination of the sample.

VN7.17
VN7.24

5. Equipment and supplies required:

Clippers
2ml sterile syringe
21g (green) sterile needle
EDTA (Ethylene Diamine Tetra-Acetic acid) blood sample bottle
Micro-haematocrit capillary tubes
Cristaseal
Hawksley micro-haematocrit centrifuge and reader
Tissue

VN7.13
Scope C (ii), (iii), (iv) & (v)

6. Preparation of equipment

I gathered all the equipment required and placed it where it was easily accessible.
I switched the centrifuge on, opened the lid and unscrewed the metal plate.
I placed the needle on the syringe.

85

7. Collection of sample:

Basil was restrained by another veterinary nurse and under the supervision of the veterinary surgeon I took the blood sample from the left jugular vein.

I placed the blood sample into an EDTA blood sample bottle, first removing the needle, and making sure I filled the bottle to the 'fill-line'. I then inverted the bottle a number of times to mix the blood with the anticoagulant to prevent the sample clotting.

I then labelled the sample bottle clearly with the name of the owner and the cat, the date and the computer reference number to identify the sample.

Vn7.3 3,4 & 5 Scope A(I), C(I) & D(I)

Date(s) sample collected and test carried out: ...23/03/04...........

8. Preparation of sample for testing/storage and preservation, prior to dispatch:

The test was performed in-house straight away. The sample was mixed thoroughly immediately prior to the test.

If there was a delay the sample would have been stored in the fridge but allowed to warm up to room temperature before testing.

VN7.3 Scope B(I)

9. Procedure(s) for test OR packaging and postage – method of dispatch (see guidance notes):

I mixed the sample thoroughly by inverting the sample bottle several times.

I dipped one end of a micro-haematocrit capillary tube into the blood and inclined it at 45 degrees to allow the blood to three quarter fill the tube by capillary action.

Holding the tube horizontally I wiped the outside of the tube with a tissue.

The unfilled end of the tube was then sealed with cristaseal and placed in the centrifuge sealed end outwards.

The same procedure was used to fill a second capillary tube, which was then placed in the centrifuge diametrically opposite the first tube to balance the samples.

I then screwed down the metal plate, closed the centrifuge and spun the samples at 10,000 revs/minute for 5 minutes.

VN7.4 3

Scope A(I), B(I), C(Iv), D(I)

Once the centrifuge had stopped spinning I removed one of the samples and read the PCV on the micro–
haematocrit reader, which has a linear scale.

To do this I placed the capillary tube in the groove on the plastic slide. I lined up the bottom of the blood with the zero line and the top of the plasma with the 100 line. I then adjusted the silver line so that it just touched the top of the column of red blood cells and read the PCV off where the silver line crossed the scale on the right hand side of the reader.

I then read the value of the other capillary tube and determined the average value.

I then recorded the results on the patient's records.

VN 7.4.6

| 10. Results of test: | The PCV was 17% |
| 11. Normal ranges: | Feline 24–45% |

12. Examples of conditions which may give rise to abnormal ranges:

A decrease in PCV is found in various types of anaemia eg haemolytic, haemorrhagic and aplastic.
An increase in PCV is seen in cases of dehydration leading to haemoconcentration eg severe diabetes mellitus, chronic nephritis, prolonged vomiting and diarrhoea.

13. Possible reasons for inaccurate results:

Haemolysis of the sample due to faulty collection including application of too much suction when taking the sample, insufficient anticoagulant, failure to mix the sample and vigorous shaking of the sample.
Failure to fill the capillary tube sufficiently.
Leakage or loss of the seal in the capillary tube.
Failure to balance the samples.
Inaccuracy reading the results.
If I had thought the results were inaccurate for any reason I would have informed the veterinary surgeon.

VN 7.4.5

Student VN's comments and signature:

Comments:

A PCV is a rapid and fairly easy test to perform and can help to identify anaemia. I now feel quite confident performing this procedure accurately.

The evidence in this log sheet is a true account of the case/procedures described and my involvement therein. The work undertaken in compiling the log is my own.

Student Veterinary Nurse's Signature: .... *Ben Gall* ....

Note – This is an example of a case log prior to evaluation, hence the absence of the Assessor Statement Box with the
Assessor signature, qualifications and date.

Example 2

LOG SHEET 6a - LABORATORY & DIAGNOSTIC AIDS

Student Veterinary Nurse's Name:		Ben Gall	VN Enrolment No:		F62195	
1. Case Details:	Species:	Feline	**Age:**	3 yrs 5 mths	**Sex:**	Male
	Breed:	Domestic Shorthair	**Weight:**	4.8 kg		
2. Case No. Identification:		Lab 6a1(Computer reference 44192) Basil. (Cross referenced to Lab 6a2)			**Assessor's Comments:**	

3. Type of procedure and reason for test:

Basil had been seen by the veterinary surgeon on previous occasions and she was becoming increasingly concerned about his deteriorating condition. She suspected that he might be suffering from Feline Infectious Anaemia (FIA). To confirm this she requested a blood sample to be taken and a full blood profile to be performed including a Pack Cell Volume (PCV) estimation. She also requested that a Leishman stained blood smear be examined for evidence of the presence of Haemobartonella felis, the causal agent of FIA and to look at the blood picture. (Cross referenced to Lab 6a2).

VN7.1 Scope A(i) (Cat)
B(i) (Blood)

4. Preparation of animal and pre-test procedures:

I accessed Basil's computer records to confirm his case records and the procedure requested by the veterinary surgeon. I also checked the consent form to ensure that he had not been fed after 8 00pm the previous evening and had not had access to water from 7 30am that morning as this could affect the blood tests. The procedure was performed in the prep room which was well lit and ventilated by air conditioning. It was also relatively quiet to reduce any distress to Basil that could have been caused by excessive noise.

Assisted by another nurse I clipped a small area of fur from the ventral aspect of the cat's neck over the left jugular vein. The area was then cleaned with chlorhexidine (Hibiscrub) 1:20 solution and swabbed with spirit to prevent the introduction of infection and possible contamination of the sample.

VN7.1.1
VN7.2.1 Scope A(i), C(i)
VN7.2.2
VN7.2.7 Scope D(i), (iii), & (v)
VN7.1.7
VN7.2.4

5. Equipment and supplies required:

Following our practice procedure for taking a blood sample and performing a PCV I provided the following items.

Laboratory coat

Disposable gloves

Clippers with a size 40 blade

2ml sterile syringe

21 g (green) needle

EDTA (Ethylene Diamine Tetra–Acetic acid) blood sample bottle

VN7.1.3 Scope C (ii), (iii), (vi) and (v)

Micro–haematocrit capillary tubes

Cristaseal

Hawksey micro–haematocrit centrifuge and reader

Tissue

Chlorhexidine solution and spirit

Cotton wool swabs.

I checked with the veterinary surgeon that I had provided all the required equipment. — VN7.1 2

6. Preparation of equipment

I gathered all the equipment and checked them to ensure they were clean/sterile and in working condition as appropriate. If any item was not fit to use I would have replaced it or reported the problem to the veterinary surgeon as appropriate. I placed the equipment for taking the sample on a disinfected surface (Trigene diluted at a ratio of 1:200) close to hand. I placed the needle on the syringe leaving it capped.

In the laboratory I switched the centrifuge on, opened the lid and unscrewed the metal plate. I prepared the rest of the laboratory equipment leaving it ready for use. — VN7.1 6, 7 & 8

7. Collection of sample:

Basil was restrained by another veterinary nurse (See Appendix 3 Restraint of a cat for jugular venipuncture) whilst I took the blood sample from the left jugular vein under the supervision of the veterinary surgeon. Basil was quite weak so needed minimal restraint. I reassured him throughout the procedure to prevent him becoming distressed and stressed. — VN7.2 & 4 Scope B(i), C(i); VN7.3 1 & 2; VN7.2 6

I placed the blood sample into an EDTA blood sample bottle, first removing the needle, and making sure I filled the bottle to the 'fill-line'. I then inverted the bottle several times to mix the blood with the anticoagulant to prevent the sample clotting.

I then labelled the sample bottle clearly with the name of the owner and the cat, the date and the computer reference number to identify the sample. — VN7.3 3, 4 & 5 Scope A(i); C(i); D(i) (Cat)

Date(s) sample collected and test carried out: .... 23-03-04 ....

8. Preparation of sample for testing/storage and preservation, prior to dispatch:	
The test was performed in house straight away. The sample was mixed thoroughly immediately prior to the test. If there was a delay the sample would have been stored in the fridge but allowed to warm up to room temperature before testing.	*VN7.3 Scope B'(i)*
9. Procedure(s) for test OR packaging and postage – method of dispatch (see guidance notes):	
I put on a lab coat and a pair of disposable gloves. I read the sample bottle label and confirmed it was the correct sample.	*VN7.4 1*
I mixed the sample thoroughly by inverting the sample bottle several times.	
I dipped one end of a Micro-haematocrit capillary tube into the blood and inclined it at 45 degrees to allow the blood to three quarter fill the tube by capillary action.	
Holding the tube horizontally I wiped the outside of the tube with a tissue.	
The unfilled end of the tube was then sealed with cristaseal and placed in the centrifuge sealed end outwards.	*VN7.4 2, 3 & 4*
The same procedure was used to fill a second capillary tube, which was then placed in the centrifuge diametrically opposite the first tube to balance the samples.	*Scope A(i)* *B(i)* *C(iv)* *D(i)*
I then screwed down the metal plate, closed the centrifuge and spun the samples at 10,000 revs/minute for 5 minutes.	
Once the centrifuge had stopped spinning I removed one of the samples and read the PCV on the micro–haematocrit reader, which has a linear scale.	
To do this I placed the capillary tube in the groove on the plastic slide. I lined up the bottom of the blood with the zero line and the top of the plasma with the 100 line. I then adjusted the silver line so that it just touched the top of the column of red blood cells and read the PCV off where the silver line crossed the scale on the right hand side of the reader.	
I then read the value of the other capillary tube and determined the average value.	*VN7.4 6*
I then recorded the results on the patient's records.	*VN7.3 7 VN7.4, 9 & 10*
I disposed of the surplus and waste materials according to practice protocol (Ref Appendix 3 Disposal of Waste).	

10. Results of test:	The PCV was 17%
11. Normal ranges:	Feline 24–45%

12. Examples of conditions which may give rise to abnormal ranges:

A decrease in PCV is found in various types of anaemia eg haemolytic, haemorrhagic and aplastic.
An increase in PCV is seen in cases of dehydration leading to haemoconcentration eg severe diabetes mellitus, chronic nephritis, prolonged vomiting and diarrhoea.

13. Possible reasons for inaccurate results:

Haemolysis of the sample due to faulty collection including application of too much suction when taking the sample, insufficient anticoagulant, failure to mix the sample and vigorous shaking of the sample.
Failure to fill the capillary tube sufficiently.
Leakage or loss of the seal in the capillary tube.
Failure to balance the samples.
Inaccuracy reading the results.
If I had thought the results were inaccurate for any reason I would have informed the veterinary surgeon.

VN7.45

Student VN's comments and signature:

Comments:

A PCV is a rapid and fairly easy test to perform and along with other tests helps to identify anaemia. I now feel quite confident performing this procedure accurately. A blood smear was also performed on the sample to look at the blood cells and also to see if there was any evidence of Haemobartonella felis as the Veterinary Surgeon suspected Basil was suffering from FIA. Unfortunately this was confirmed.

The evidence in this log sheet is a true account of the case/procedures described and my involvement therein. The work undertaken in compiling the log is my own.

Student Veterinary Nurse's Signature: .... Ben Gall ....

Note – This is an example of a case log prior to evaluation, hence the absence of the Assessor Statement Box with the Assessor signature, qualifications and date.

92

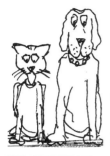

Chapter 5

Cross-referencing

Cross-referencing can be an important tool in compiling a concise yet comprehensive portfolio. To achieve this it is vital that the concept of cross-referencing is properly understood and that it is used appropriately.

Students often have difficulty seeing further than individual case logs, and fail to appreciate the wider concept of the portfolio as a whole. The building blocks of the portfolio are indeed the logs, which build into individual modules, which in turn make up the portfolio.

To consider an analogy, cast your mind back to one of your first anatomy lessons: you were taught a similar concept that cells are the basic building blocks of the body, which build into tissues, which in turn make up the body. Just as a damaged liver can affect the health of an animal, poor and inaccurate case logs can have a detrimental effect on the quality of your portfolio.

The benefits of cross-referencing include:

* A reduction in the number of clinical cases that need to be found, as one clinical case presented at the surgery may lend itself to providing potential case log material for more than one module.

- A diminution in the size of your portfolio while at the same time providing the necessary evidence of your competence. Remember, your portfolio is not evaluated by weight but by content!

- Allowing you to provide more evidence of competence than an individual case log allows.

Level 2

Cross-referencing is actively encouraged in the portfolio module guidance notes at Level 2. Table 5.1 gives examples of scenarios when cross-referencing could be a useful tool.

Table 5.1 Level 2 cross-referencing opportuniites

Scenario	Cross-referencing opportunity
Module 3 Admit and discharge animals 3b – Discharge animals after verterinary treatment	*Module 2* Reception and client support 2b – Dispensing medication to clients
Module 4 Prepare for and assist with medical veterinary procedures and investigations	*Module 5* Basic nursing. 5b – Basic first aid
Module 5 Basic nursing 5a – Basic animal management	*Module 5* Basic nursing 5c – Administration of medication

The latter example is illustrated in case logs 5a and 5c.

Level 3

Level 3 modules provide a wealth of opportunities to utilise a clinical case in a variety of logs. Table 5.2 gives examples of clinical cases and their cross-referencing potential.

Note that this list is not exhaustive but rather indicative of cross-referencing opportunities.

Table 5.2 Clinical cases and cross-referencing potential

Clinical case	Cross-referencing potential
Pyometra	Modules 6, 7 and 9 or 10
Road traffic accident involving a fracture	Modules 8 and 9 or 10
Mammary tumour	Modules 6, 7, 8 and 9 or 10
Ruptured cruciate ligament	Modules 8 and 9 or 10
Urolithiasis	Modules 6, 7, 8 and 9 or 10
Diabetes mellitus	Modules 6 and 7
Renal failure	Modules 6 and 7, including fluid therapy
Splenic tumour	Modules 6 and 7, including fluid therapy, 8 including ultrasound and 9 or 10

Handy hints

* Critically appraise clinical cases with a view to their cross-referencing potential.

* Ensure the cross-referencing is appropriate and will add to the evidence of your competence in the portfolio.

* Consider the practicality of cross-referencing certain modules, for instance Module 9 – Surgical nursing and theatre practice with Module 10 – Anaesthesia, this is not acceptable as you will not be able to adequately cover the occupational standards.

* Ensure that you indicate clearly in all the case logs cross-referenced that you have done so in the case identification box and the individual boxes of the relevant logs (see case log examples 5a and 5c).

* Indicate all cross-references on the portfolio contents page.

LOG SHEET 5a - BASIC ANIMAL MANAGEMENT

Student Veterinary Nurse's Name:		Sheila Tzu	VN Enrolment No:		E 19522	
1. Case Details:	**Species:**	Canine	**Age:**	5 months	**Sex:**	Male
	Breed:	Cross breed	**Weight:**	8.2 Kg		
2. Case Number – identification:		BAM 5 Client ref: 1452 Cross reference to log AMA 2	Assessor's Comments:			

3. Reason for hospitalisation:

The patient was admitted by the Veterinary Surgeon for suspected fractured pelvis following a road traffic accident the previous evening. Tommy was to be nursed and observed for the day then kept in overnight in order to be confined and X-rayed the following day.

4. Type of accommodation and bedding material used, to include: any relevant environmental factors

- Accommodation – a medium sized kennel. See Appendix 1 – animal accommodation. I chose this size because it wasn't too big and provided him with the necessary confinement. This was essential to prevent him moving too much and damaging his fractured pelvis and surrounding tissues even more.
- A double layer of Vet bed was provided for warmth and comfort and thickness to help to prevent pressure sores which may have occurred due to his lack of movement and contact with the hard surface of the kennel.
- I covered him with a light blanket for warmth because he wasn't moving around and producing his own heat.

5. Accommodation cleaning protocol, to include: type of disinfectant, dilution of, mechanical cleaning procedures, frequency of cleaning and disposal of waste:

- The kennel was prepared and cleaned as required and all waste was disposed of in clinical waste – ref Appendix 3 – Cleaning Protocols.
- Tommy could not get up to pass urine and he was initially incontinent so his Vetbed had to be changed regularly. Each time it was soiled it was washed separately in the washing machine and dried in the dryer.

96

6. Feeding Regime:

No food was given on the first day as Tommy was to have a general anaesthetic and x-ray the following morning. He was offered water and drank a small amount at first (about 40ml) but didn't seem to want any water later. His water bowl was removed at 8.00am on the morning of his G/A.

3 hours after recovery from anaesthetic he drank readily so it was then decided to offer him a small amount (1 quarter of a can, mixed with warm water) of canned Hills i/d. This is a balanced diet which is easy to digest for a patient following a general anaesthetic. It is also quite palatable and Tommy appeared very hungry.

We continued to feed him a quarter of a can at 4 hour intervals – see hospitalisation form.

7. Nursing care and monitoring of the animal: Please give details of grooming, wound management, cleaning, monitoring of vital signs and "TLC".

- Tommy's vital signs were monitored 3 times a day but all was normal from when he was first admitted until discharge 2 days later – see hospitalisation form. Initially his respiratory rate was slightly raised at 30BPM (15–30 BPM – breaths per minute normal) but this was probably due to his severe pain in the pelvic area.

- He was given plenty of TLC to try to comfort him and to distract him from the pain. I gently washed his face with damp cotton wool but did not groom him as his coat was very short and his caudal end was so painful.

- The evening following his x-ray and the following morning, I gently encouraged him to stand then turned him over to ensure that too much pressure wasn't applied to any particular pressure points such as his damaged pelvis, hocks or elbows.

Date(s) specify duration of hospitalisation Admitted ....15-03-04...........
                                              X-ray ....16-03-04...........
                                              Discharged ....17-03-04...........

8. Medication administered: (details can be cross referenced to Log 5c)

Apart from the general anaesthetic, intramuscular pain killing injections of Vetergesic (Buphrenorphine – 0.25 ml) were administered every 12 hours by myself or the Vet. **Cross reference AMA 2.**

Student's comments, to include: the part the student has played in this case:

Comments:
The X-ray confirmed that the patient had a fracture of his pubic symphysis. The vet advised that the best treatment was confinement and rest. Tommy is a young dog so this type of fracture should repair quite quickly.
My role in this case was to make the patient as comfortable as possible as he was initially in a lot of pain. I spent a lot of time gently turning him from left to right recumbency until he was finally able to move himself by the time he went home.
I was also asked to observe and note his bladder and bowel function to ensure that there was no underlying nerve damage.
This was a very rewarding case and very satisfying when Tommy came in for his check earlier today. He walked in wagging his tail and licked my hand – I like think that this was in appreciation of his TLC!

Copy of hospitalisation record attached   YES ☒   NO ☐

The evidence in this log sheet is a true account of the case/procedures described and my involvement therein. The work undertaken in compiling the log is my own.

Student veterinary nurse's signature   ... *Sheila Tzu* ....

Note – This is an example of a case log prior to evaluation, hence the absence of the Assessor Statement Box with the Assessor signature, qualifications and date.

LOG SHEET 5c – ADMINISTRATION OF MEDICATION TO ANIMALS

Student Veterinary Nurse's Name:		Sheila Tzu	VN Enrolment No:		E 19522	
1. Case Details:	**Breed:**	Cross breed	**Weight:**	8.2 Kgs	**Sex:**	Male
	Species:	Canine	**Age:**	5 months		
2. Case Number – identification:		AMA2(Client Record 1452) Cross Reference to Log BAM 5	**3. Date Administered:** ......15 March 2004			
4. Name of medication administered, to include trade & generic names and classification and drug form: e.g. antibiotic/cream, sedative/injection etc.			**Assessor's Comments:**			

Trade name – Vetergesic

Generic name – Buphrenorphine. Contains 0.3mg/ml

Classification –POM (Prescription Only Medicine – can only be prescribed by a Veterinary Surgeon for an animal in their care) Controlled drug, Schedule 3

Drug form – Analgesic (pain killer). Injection.

5. Dose details

Dose Rate:

0.3 –0.6 ml / 10Kg

May be repeated every 12 hours if necessary.

Dose given (including calculation):

Dose rate per Kg = $\frac{0.3}{10}$ = 0.03ml   So – Dose rate = 0.03 × 8.2(Weight of patient in kgs) = 0.246ml

On the instructions of the Vet – 0.25ml was to be administered

6. Reason for administration, basic effect of the drug and how it was administered: The patient had a suspected pelvic fracture **Cross Ref: BAM 5** and the Buprenorphine would provide fast, effective and long lasting pain relief. The drug was to be administered via intramuscular injection as the preferred route because it would be faster acting than subcutaneously. It would begin to act in 15–20 minutes. The trapezius muscle in the back of the neck was chosen instead of the quadriceps in the hind leg because the patient was in a great deal of pain in its pelvic area. I checked all of the patient's details and then confirmed the drug and dose with the Veterinary Surgeon. I used a 1ml syringe because it is easier to measure a small amount and a 25g 5/8" needle as a fine gauge would be less painful. Another nurse gently restrained the dog while I gave the injection. I parted the hair at the back of the neck and swabbed the area with spirit. I inserted the needle at a 90° angle and withdrew on the plunger to ensure that I had not punctured a blood vessel. I then quickly injected the drug, withdrew the needle and then massaged the area.	
7. Health & Safety issues and precautions taken: *If a controlled drug, specify the recording and storage requirements and attach a copy of the register entry if applicable.* The syringe and needle were disposed of in the clinical waste sharps box. After withdrawing the drug from the bottle I replaced the needle cap until the injection was given. This was to prevent accidental injection of anyone. Vetergesic is a Schedule 3 controlled drug which means that it must be securely stored in a locked cupboard (only the Vets have keys) and records of its purchase must be kept by the Practice principal. Unlike Schedule 2 drugs, its use does not need to be entered in the controlled drugs register.	

Student's Comments and Signature:

Comments:

I recorded the details of the drug administration on the patient's hospital record and also on the computer case record.

The administration of the drug did seem quite painful for the patient just at the time of injection but I was very pleased how quickly the pain killer began to work. The dog was much calmer and soon settled down to sleep.

The evidence in this log sheet is a true account of the case/procedures described and my involvement therein. The work undertaken in compiling the log is my own.

Student veterinary nurse's signature: *Sheila Tzu* ....

Note – This is an example of a case log prior to evaluation, hence the absence of the Assessor Statement Box with the Assessor signature, qualifications and date.

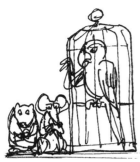

Chapter 6

Spot the deliberate mistakes

Included here are two very poor case logs. Spot the deliberate mistakes, then check the following bullet points for ways of drastically improving the evidence and demonstrate your knowledge and understanding, as well as inadvertently covering many of the standards without having realised it!

See Log sheet 5b

See Log sheet 3b

LOGSHEET 5b – BASIC FIRST AID

Student Veterinary Nurse's Name:		Danny Dimwit	VN Enrolment No:		
1. Case Details:	**Species:**	Cat	**Age:**	Old	**Sex:** Female
	Breed:	Domestic	**Weight:**	7 pounds	
2. Case Number – identification:		BFA 2 (Computer Ref: 01–04–03 – 13)	**Assessor's Comments:**		

3. History:

The cat was brought down to the surgery without an appointment, as it was unable to breath. The owner thought that she had been hit by a car.

4. Clinical evaluation of patient:

The cat was collapsed and shocked. She was blue and her CRT (capillary refill time) was more than 5 seconds. She was having difficulty breathing (dysnoea) and her respiratory rate was very irregular. She was gasping for air. The patient was also very cold.

5. First aid emergency procedure carried out:

The Veterinary Surgeon obtained a consent form from the owner, while I admitted the cat and as directed by the Vet proceeded to make an oxygen tent.

I placed the cat in a wire cat carrier and covered it with clingfilm. I then connected the oxygen pipe from the oxygen cylinder into the carrier. I turned the oxygen dial to 3 litres per minute. This allowed an oxygen rich environment to hopefully reduce the cat's respiratory distress.

I put the carrier on the top of a heat pad to help to raise her temperature.

6. Monitoring of the animal:

I observed the cat from the outside of the cage and monitored it regularly.

It was a little distressed at first but then became more comfortable.

As instructed by the Vet I then moved the cat to a hospitalisation cage. I gave it fleece bedding for comfort and warmth and a litter tray. I also gave the patient a bowl of water.

The front of the cage was covered with a thick towel, to keep the cat calm and quiet. I continually observed the cat's breathing and recorded the findings on the hospitalisation sheet.

7. Outcome of first aid emergency treatment:

Even though the cat's breathing initially seemed to improve while it was in the oxygen tank, but then it's condition gradually deteriorated throughout the day.

The Owners did not want an X-ray and decided to have the cat put to sleep.

8. Dates to include: date of incident and full timescale range, if appropriate	01-04-04 - 9.25am to 9.50pm in oxygen tent 3.00pm euthanased

Students comments, to include confirmation of your role in the procedures and any additional detail not given previously:

Comments:

I was relieved that the Veterinary Surgeon was present for this case. She examined the patient, whilst I pinned her to the table. I now feel more confident about administering oxygen to a distressed patient, but would always check with the receptionist first. The cat was quite old and it was a pity that the owners decided on euthanasia, later in the day.

The evidence in this log sheet is a true account of the case/procedures described and my involvement therein. The work undertaken in compiling the log is my own.

Student Veterinary Nurse's signature .... *D. Dinmont* ....

Assessor's Comments:

The procedures and details recorded within this log sheet have been observed by myself / a witness* (witness name ....)
and have been carried out correctly and competently. *please delete

Comments:

Assessor's signature: ....   Assessor's name: ....

Assessor's qualifications: ....   Date: ....15th May 2004 ....

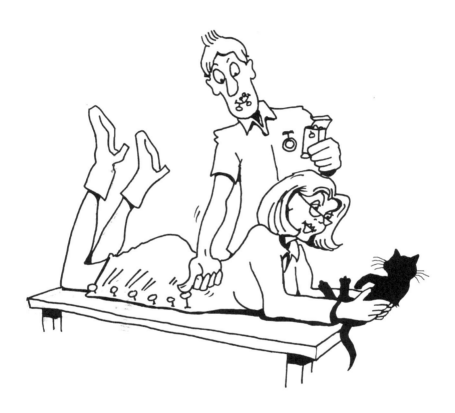

"She examined the patient, whilst I pinned her to the table."

Logsheet 5b – Basic first aid

☸ VN Enrolment Number omitted.

1 Case details

☸ Species – use correct terms where known, ie feline.

☸ Age – give an approximation if unknown.

☸ Weight – always use kilograms, or both kilograms and pounds.

☸ Sex – state neuter status, whether known or not.

☸ Breed – state whether long or short-haired.

2 Case number – identification

☸ Date of computer reference does not match with date the case was seen as in Box 8.

3 History

☸ What is meant by *unable to breathe?* Was it asphyxiating, dead, or just having difficulty?

☸ Who was involved in the RTA? The owner or the cat?

☸ Do we know how long ago the RTA occurred? Time is very relevant in most first-aid cases.

4 Clinical evaluation of patient

☸ *Shocked* should be explained.

☸ What was *blue?* The cat's mucous membranes or its coat colour? You should explain what the implication of cyanosis, is eg a lack of oxygen because it was having difficulty breathing.

☸ Normal CRT is < 2 seconds. A patient with a CRT of ·5 seconds would probably be dead! Always state the normal so that abnormalities are clear.

* Terminology spelling mistake – dyspnoea.

* What was the respiratory rate?

* What was *cold?* Was it her extremities that actually felt cold? State whether you took her temperature, and if so what was the reading? State the normal in order to demonstrate any abnormality.

5 First-aid emergency procedure carried out

* What was covered with clingfilm? The cat or the carrier?

6 Monitoring of the animal

* What did you observe about the patient?

* What was monitored, and how often?

* How was the vet informed of any changes?

* Describe how you knew that the cat was *more comfortable.*

* How could the cat's breathing be continually observed if the cage was covered with a thick towel?

* What findings were recorded? A copy of the hospitalisation form could be included, highlighting your input.

7 Outcome of first-aid emergency treatment

* Spelling mistake – oxygen tank/tent.

* Poor use of grammar.

8 Dates to include:

* Times not correct – was it am or pm?

Student's Comments and signature

* Who was *pinned to the table?* The patient or the vet?

Explain how the patient was restrained. It was obviously distressed and so required very careful and gentle handling.

- Is the receptionist qualified veterinary personnel, experienced enough to advice a student?

- Signature does not match student's name.

Assessor date

- More than two weeks have elapsed since the evidence occurred. You are expected to write up your case logs within a few days of the evidence occurring. You should then present this to your assessor for correction, and for the assessor to include any questions required in order to check your underpinning knowledge. The log should then be signed off by your assessor within two weeks, or they should explain in the comments section why it was not.

Student Veterinary Nurse's Name:		April Foolish	VN Enrolment No:	F729113	
1. Case Details:	Species:	Lagomorph	Age:	10 mths	Sex: F
	Breed:	English Flop	Weight:	20 kg	Client Type:
2. Case Number – identification:		Discharge 1	Assessor's Comments:		

3. Veterinary procedure carried out:

The rabbit was admitted for the removal of an identification ring on its leg.

4. Date & time animal discharged: ...... 1/4/04 ....   **5. Date & time of next appointment:** ....

6. Describe any preparation of the animal prior to discharge:

I checked the rabbit had recovered from the anaesthetic by rattling the bars on its cage, it jumped so I knew it was awake.

I carried the rabbit through to the waiting room and gave it to its owner together with its medication.

7. Information and advice given to the client:

I gave the client an information sheet on the post operative care of the rabbit and instructed her to read it.

I booked her an appointment for a check up.

8. State any medication or treatment (s) supplied to owner:*	YES ☑ NO ☐

Comments:

I gave the antibiotic solution to the owner and told her the instructions were quite simple and were printed on the label.

Details can be cross referenced to dispensing logs

9. Was the method for administrating any medication or treatment(s) to the animal demonstrated to the owner?	YES ☐ NO ☑

Comments:

Student's Comments and Signature:

Comments:

I was quiet nervous about this discharge as it was the first one I had done on my own. The rabbit did struggle a bit in the waiting room especially when I gave the client her medication but I thought overall it went well.

The evidence in this log sheet is a true account of the case/procedures described and my involvement therein. The work undertaken in compiling the log is my own.

Student veterinary nurse's signature ....

Note – This is an example of a case log prior to evaluation, hence the absence of the *Assessor Statement* Box with the Assessor signature, qualifications and date.

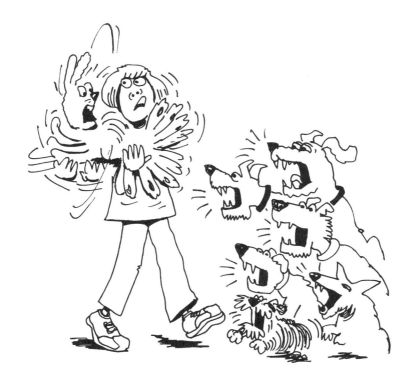

"The rabbit did struggle a bit in the waiting room."

Logsheet 3b – Discharge after veterinary treatment

1 Case details

* Species – Strictly speaking, a lagomorph is not a species but an order of animal classification, including rabbits and hares. It is more appropriate to use rabbit or the Latin equivalent *Oryctolagus cuniculus.*

  Another area of confusion often encountered concerns guinea pigs. Frequently, where the subject is a guinea pig the student fills in the species box as a rodent. A rodent is not a species. The species is guinea pig or cavy.

* English Flop is a careless mistake and should of course read Lop. Take care with spelling.

* Weight 20 kg – obviously another careless mistake, or 'Floppy' has a serious weight problem. This could have disastrous consequences if this weight was used to calculate a drug dosage: Imagine if it was used to calculate an anaesthetic dose!

* Client Type omitted. Always include this if appropriate in the case log, ie Current, new, young, elderly or with special needs, as this can affect your approach to the case.

2 Case Number – identification

No computer reference number. If at all possible it is important to include this to aid identification of the cases.

3 Veterinary procedure carried out

* Lacking important details.

* Which leg?

* Why did the identification ring need removing?

4 Date and time animal discharged

1/04/04. Quite appropriate in this case!

5 Date and time of next appointment

Omitted. This must always be indicated even if no appointment is necessary.

6 Describe any preparation of the animal prior to discharge

This is an example of how not to prepare an animal for discharge. Not a single performance criterion is covered in this section! Look at Element VN 6.3 in the occupational standards to see how this aspect of the log could be improved.

7 Information and advice given to the client

Or, in this case, lack of information. It is important to demonstrate your competence regarding informing the client of how to care for their animal post-operatively, and how to seek advice if they are worried. Luckily, April booked the client an appointment for a check-up and gave her the medication she needed! See Student Comments and Signature. Be careful to write exactly what you mean.

8 State any medication or treatment(s) supplied to the owner

Be specific. Remember this is an opportunity to cross-reference these details to the dispensing case logs.

9 Was the method for administering any medication or treatment(s) demonstrated to the owner?

A golden opportunity was missed to satisfy VN 5.3 5.

Student Comments and Signature

Spelling of quiet instead of quite. You must take care with spelling and grammar. No student signature. It is vital that you sign every case log to prove that it is your own work and that it is a true account of the case. However, reading this case log and the student comments, it is little wonder that she has not signed it! The assessor comments could also prove both illuminating and interesting reading.

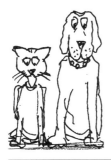

Chapter 7

What if?

We are constantly being asked for advice on various aspects of portfolio compilation. This chapter is designed to try and answer some of the most frequently asked questions.

This list of What if? questions is not exhaustive, but hopefully will provide valuable information to help you.

What if:

I am not happy with an assessment decision?

There is an appeals procedure, which you can use. Briefly, the first port of call is your assessor. If you are still not satisfied by the outcome then you can appeal to your internal verifier, and finally to your external verifier. Details of the procedure are available from the RCVS.

I am working at a branch surgery: Will this count towards my hours?

Provided the branch surgery is an approved practice, ie a TP, then the hours will count. You must of course have access to your assessor for a minimum of two days a week.

I have not completed 60% of my portfolio by the time I intend to enter for the RCVS examination?

You will not be able to enter for the examination, as your practice principal has to certify that you have completed 60% of your portfolio by the time you enter. You will have to enter for the examination at the next opportunity, provided you have completed 60% of the portfolio when you apply.

At my practice we send of most of the laboratory samples to a commercial laboratory?

This will make completion of Module 6 – Laboratory and diagnostic aids difficult to complete. The solution is for your assessor, in collaboration with the internal verifier, to arrange a secondment to a practice where you can undertake the necessary training to enable you to satisfy the occupational standards. A similar situation could also be encountered:

* if the number of radiographs taken per week is not sufficient,

* if your practice does not have ultrasound or endoscopy facilities

* or if you work for a charity TP where payment is not taken.

My portfolio is lost?

Calamity!! You must keep a photocopy of your portfolio, as if the original is lost for any reason all your efforts and evidence of competence will be lost. It is not sufficient just to keep a copy on disk, as this will not have your assessor's signature or extra questions on it.

I fail to prove competence during an assessment?

Do not worry, your assessor will negotiate another assessment opportunity and will give you feedback as to why you failed this time.

My assessor leaves the practice?

If there is another assessor in the practice, and provided they do not have too many students, they could take you under their care. However, if the assessor's leaving results in the practice not having an assessor, this may be a serious situation and can have serious consequences for your training. The practice must inform the VNAC of the situation as a priority, and your internal verifier, in conjunction with your practice, will attempt to resolve the situation. If an assessor is not in place then the VNAC will suspend the practice, which will mean that you cannot continue your training until there is an assessor or a student assessor in place.

My assessor is only a student assessor?

This should present no problems provided that arrangements are made for your assessor's decisions to be countersigned by a qualified assessor. This could be an assessor in your practice, at a neighbouring practice, or at your VNAC.

I hardly seem to see my assessor and I am finding it difficult to complete my portfolio?

Contact with your assessor is very important and should be an absolute minimum of two days a week. If this is not the case, in the first instance you should have a word with your assessor to try and resolve the issue, and then with the practice principal. If this fails then consult your internal verifier, who will be able to resolve the problem.

I do not get any help to improve my knowledge and understanding to enable me to pass my RCVS examinations and complete my portfolio?

Students who attend any sort of formal course must also receive tutorials within the TP of at least three hours per week. Where training is provided entirely within the TP this should be a minimum of seven hours per week. These sessions need not be continuous as one session, but can be spread throughout the week, but all contact should be recorded.

I have completed my Level two portfolio but failed my RCVS Level two written examinations: Can I start to complete my Level 3 portfolio?

This is not recommended by the RCVS as it is felt that collecting Level 3 evidence could jeopardise your Level 2 progress. However, there may be instances where commencing collection of evidence may be acceptable. If in doubt, contact your internal verifier or the RCVS website under Frequently Asked Questions.

I change my job and move to a different practice?

Ensure that the new practice is a TP, and then the process is quite simple. You need to complete the RCVS Annex Ciii Notification of Student Change of Employment and/or Centre and send this off to the RCVS. The principals of the current and receiving practices must sign the form. Failure to notify to the RCVS of a change of TP or VNAC can result in loss of recordable training time.

I do not have access to a computer to complete my portfolio?

This is not a problem. You can handwrite the case logs, but make sure they are legible.

My assessor leaves and has not signed the authentication form?

This is a difficult situation and can be easily avoided if any contributors to the portfolio sign the Portfolio Signature Authentication Sheet (Annex D) immediately they first sign off a case log. If this is not done and the person leaves the practice then you will have to track them down and obtain their signature. If this is not possible the relevant case logs will not be acceptable. Hence the importance of keeping the RCVS annexes current!

I am having difficulty obtaining a first-aid case?

This is one of the few occasions when a simulation is acceptable. The fact that the case log is a simulation should be made clear. However, where simulations are used these should properly reflect the requirements of real working situations to be acceptable.

I have a really good case but it involves a wildlife patient?

The Veterinary Nursing Occupational Standards define an exotic as 'Small pets other than cats and dogs, and may include birds, rabbits, reptiles, rodents and small mammals'.
The key requirement is that the animal is a pet and is therefore owned. Some students have used wildlife unrelated to the definition and have tried to include cases on zoo or marine animals, which is not acceptable as the evidence produced is unlikely to be relevant to the standards. It would be a concern if you did not have contact with exotic species during your training to enable you to complete the case logs. Secondment to another practice might be an option. Under certain circumstances an appropriate wildlife case log can be used. These can be accessed on the RCVS website under Frequently Asked Questions, along with other useful information.

I have photographs of restraining animals for various procedures: Can I include them in my portfolio?

Certainly this is valuable evidence of competence and reduces tedious repetition in the portfolio. This is also applicable to other areas demonstrating competence. Remember to authenticate any inclusions in the portfolio.

My internal verifier comes to observe an assessment with my assessor?

Don't panic: The internal verifier is assessing the assessment process, not you. They will be concentrating on the assessor. If the external verifier is also involved they will be assessing the internal verifier assessing your assessor, not you.

I am off work for a considerable time and cannot continue with my portfolio?

This can be a problem. You need to talk with your assessor, who will consult the internal verifier, who will be able to advise you on the best course of action. This might include applying for unit certification of the modules you have already completed.

I cannot cope with the workload?

Have a word with your assessor or your college tutor – they will be able to help.

When I qualify I would like to progress and develop my potential?

There are various educational opportunities available, including diploma courses and veterinary nursing degrees.

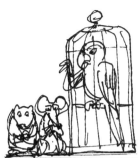

Chapter 8
Role of the assessor

The importance of the role of the assessor in the NVQ assessment process cannot be overemphasised. The assessor is pivotal to the success of the scheme.

A good assessor needs many attributes and skills to be able to perform their role, not least a sense of humour!

The responsibilities of the assessor are manifold and include:

* Being conversant with the National Occupational Standards and the Objective Syllabus and their relevance to the Portfolio.

* Providing support and advice to the student veterinary nurse (SVN). This is of paramount importance, in our view.

* Agreeing an individual assessment plan with the SVN. This plan should be regularly reviewed and revised. Accurate records of the plan should be kept and updated accordingly.

* Observing the SVN's performance in practice and judging evidence of their performance.

* Making assessment decisions against the Occupational Standards/syllabus.

☙ Providing the student with prompt, accurate and constructive feedback on their performance.

☙ Ensuring that the student's demonstration of competence is recorded appropriately.

☙ Liaising with the internal verifier and the external verifier where appropriate.

Handy hints

☙ Familiarise yourself with the National Occupational Standards and the Objective Syllabus.

☙ Ensure that the student begins completion of the RCVS Annexes as soon as they receive their portfolio, and that they update them in an ongoing manner. The Portfolio Signature Authentication annex is especially important. If a staff member has signed a case log as an assessor or a witness, and then leaves the practice before signing the authentication sheet, obtaining a signature subsequently can be a major problem.

☙ Arrange regular meetings with the student to develop an assessment plan. Record these meetings and their outcomes.

☙ Use the Occupational Standards as your bible and encourage your students to do the same. If the students consult the standards when writing up their case logs this can considerably reduce the amount of extra questioning required. Often the student has fulfilled the PC and scope requirements but has not documented the fact.

☙ Remember that once an area of the standards has been satisfactorily assessed it need not be revisited. The guidance notes at the beginning of each module are just that – a guide. It is covering the PCs and scope that demonstrate competence. If we consider Module 10 – Anaesthesia, in the guidance notes it states that six anaesthetic case logs should be completed with accompanying anaesthetic record charts. However, if the student has covered all the PCs and scope (Unit VN12) in, for example, four case logs, then there is no necessity to complete the outstanding case logs. Used appropriately, this will considerably reduce the workload of both the assessor and the student.

* Encourage the student to use a personalised copy of the Occupational Standards and to tick off the relevant PCs and scope as they are covered.

* When checking the student's case logs indicate in the Assessor Comments column the relevant PCs and scope covered. This will endear you to your internal verifier, as it makes their role much easier!

* Ensure you know the name of your internal verifier and have a contact number. Remember, they will give you help and support. Do not be apprehensive about an internal verifier visit: Treat it as a golden opportunity to discuss any queries or questions you or your student may have.

* During such a visit explain to the student that the internal verifier is observing you, not them. Often the student feels quite stressed and is afraid they are letting their assessor down. This is not the case, and the internal verifier will make this clear to the student. If you have a visit from the external verifier they will be observing the internal verifier, not the assessor or the student.

* Make sure you attend the assessor workshops arranged by your VNAC. These are occasions to meet with colleagues and to be updated on recent developments. Advice and help on various aspects of the assessment process will also be given.

* Read the RCVS *Veterinary Nursing News* and your VNAC Newsletter; both are valuable sources of information.

* Remember that all additional information included in the portfolio, eg hospitalisation charts, student appendices, anaesthetic records, etc, must have the student's name, signature, enrolment number, the assessor's signature, TDLB qualifications and the date on each sheet. Also, if the assessor is a student assessor the sheet must be countersigned by a qualified assessor, with their TDLB qualifications and the date.

* Ensure that the questions asked in the Case Log Assessor column are relevant and cover the appropriate PCs and scope.

* Following are some suggestions as to how extra PCs and scope could be covered for case logs previously covered in Chapter 4 – Cross-referencing, Dispensing medication – Jackie Russell, and Radiography – Bernard Saint.

Module 2b – Units VN1 and VN5

Chapter 4 – National occupational standards – Dispensing medication – Jackie Russell.

Dispensing medication to clients.

PCs and scope nat covered in this log
VN1.3 B(iv), (v)
VN5.1 A(i) , B(ii)
VN5.2 A(i)
VN5.3 C(i)
VN5.4 A(i)

Ideas for assessor questions to cover standards not covered by this log:

VN1.3 B(iv) and (v) – 7

Did you issue the client with a Practice receipt?

VN1.3 C(ii) – 8

How would you have dealt with the situation if the client had disagreed with the cost of the tablets?

VN 5.2A(ii) 5,7

If the client had not been happy with your recommendation to worm the dog every three months, what action would you have taken?

VN 5.3C(i) –2

Can the client expect to see any side effects from these tablets?

VN5.3C(i) 6 and 7

How should the client dispose of any unwanted medication?

Standards Module 8a (Unit VN9)

Radiography – 'Bernard Saint'.

PCs and scope not covered by this log:

9.1 Ai, Bii or Biii

Ci, Cii. Monitoring badges should be mentioned in another log, even though they have probably been referred to in the health and safety risk assessment.

Di, Ei – Question: When are cassettes cleaned, and at what point are they reloaded with film?

Dii - An appendix could be used to demonstrate how processing solutions are prepared. It must, however, be referred to in a future case log.

Ei – Question: How can cross-contamination be prevented when using foam wedges?

Eiii – Can be included in an exotic case.

Eiv – Include in an infectious case. Ev - Include in an infectious case or question about zoonoses.

9.2

Ciii – Question: What potential difficulties could have arisen during this procedure?

Civ – Include a log where there is some loss of diagnostic quality, or use questions.

Di, ii, iii, iv, v – All environmental conditions can usually be covered in an exotic case, or use questioning.

9.3

9.35 – Disposal of waste can be covered in a contrast media study, or if excrement is passed during a procedure.

Di

Dii – Question: What invalid results might sagging of the spine have had on the final image?

Diii, iv – Include in future logs or question. Both could be included in an appendix that identifies problems.

Conclusion

You as an assessor are very important in this assessment process, and although it seems difficult at times, the immense satisfaction that you feel when your student achieves VN status makes it all worthwhile. Also remember that help is at hand via your internal verifier, who is there to give you help and support.

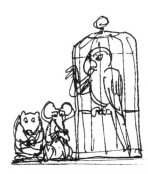

Appendix A

Useful names and addresses

British Small Animal Veterinary Association (BSAVA)
Woodrow House
1 Telford Way
Waterwells Business Park
Quedgeley
Gloucester GL2 4AB
01452 726700

British Veterinary Nursing Association (BVNA)
Suite 11, Shenval House
South Road
Harlow
Essex CM20 2BD
01279 450567

LANTRA
Lantra House
NAC
Kenilworth
Warwickshire CV8 2LG
0845 707 8007
www.lantra.co.uk

Myerscough College
Myerscough Hall
Bilsborrow
Preston
01995 642222
www.myerscough.ac.uk

Qualifications and Curriculum Authority (QCA)
83 Piccadilly
London W1J 8QA
www.qca.org.uk

Royal College of Veterinary Surgeons (RCVS)
Belgravia House
62–64 Horseferry Road
London SW1P 2AF
0207 222 2001
www.rcvs.org.uk

Scottish Qualification Authority (SQA)
Hanover House
24 Douglas Street
Glasgow G2 7 N8
020 7222 2001

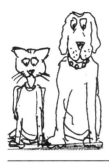

Appendix B

Further reading

LANTRA (2002) *Assessment strategy.* Lantra Connect
LANTRA (2002) *Veterinary Nursing National Occupational Standards and Qualification Structures for NVQ Levels 2 and 3.* Lantra Connect

QCA (2002) *NVQ Code of practice.* QCA Publications
QCA (2002) *Developing an assessment strategy for NVQs.* QCA Publications
These two publications are available from
QCA Publications
PO Box 99
Sudbury
Suffolk CO10 3SN
0787 884 444

RCVS (2002) *Veterinary Nurse Training Scheme. Portfolio. Small animal evidence route.* RCVS, London
RCVS (2001) *RCVS Training Centre handbook,* 3rd edn. RCVS, London
RCVS *Veterinary Nursing News.* RCVS, London
Veterinary Nursing
Veterinary Nursing Times
Veterinary Practice Nurse

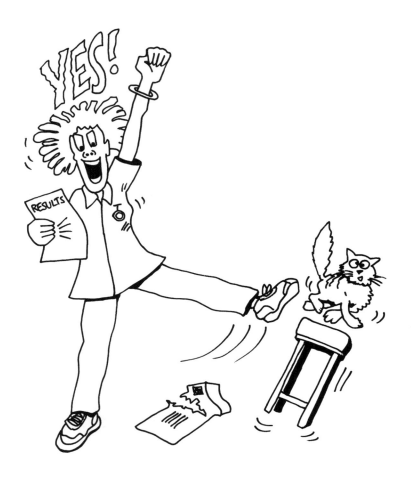

Index